Thai Herbal Medicine

Traditional Recipes for Health & Harmony

Second Edition

Other books by C. Pierce Salguero

Encyclopedia of Thai Massage,
2nd Edition

Thai Massage Workbook,
2nd edition

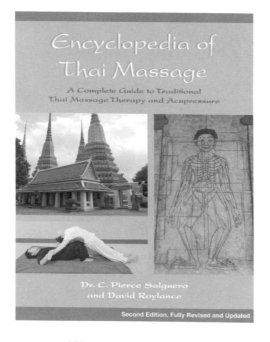

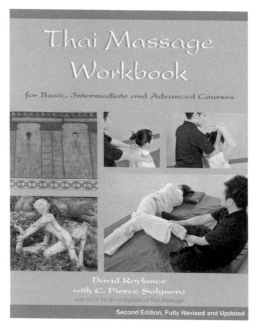

ISBN 978-1-84409-563-6

ISBN 978-1-84409-564-3

available from your local bookstore,
or directly from publisher at

www.findhornpress.com

Thai Herbal Medicine

Traditional Recipes for Health & Harmony

Nephyr Jacobsen

and

Dr. Pierce Salguero

with a contribution from

Tracy Wells

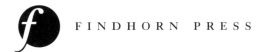

FINDHORN PRESS

First published by Findhorn Press 2003. Second edition, fully revised
and updated, published by Findhorn Press 2013.

ISBN: 978-1-84409-627-5

British Library Cataloguing-in-Publication Data.
A catalogue record for this book is available from the British Library.

Edited by Nicky Leach
Cover design by Richard Crookes
Interior design by Damian Keenan
Printed and bound in USA

Published by
Findhorn Press
117-121 High Street,
Forres IV36 1AB Scotland,
United Kingdom

t +44-(0)1309-690582
f +44(0)131-777-2711
e info@findhornpress.com
www.findhornpress.com

Important Note

This book reports on the herbal medicine recommendations made in Traditional Thai Medicine (TTM) circles. Information has been compiled from many sources including historical Thai texts, contemporary research papers, personal instruction from TTM practitioners, Thai government sources, and traditional herbal lore. Many of the herbs in this collection are well known, but in most cases the therapeutic claims made in this book have not been evaluated by the Western professional herbalist community or Western food and drug governing bodies. We strongly emphasize that use of the herbs presented in this book, especially the non-culinary ones, be undertaken only by trained herbalists, with full knowledge of local laws and at your own risk.

Please understand that this text is not meant to replace formal training with a skillful instructor in the art and practice of traditional herbal medicine, nor should it replace consultation with a properly trained doctor when choosing a remedy for yourself or others. The inherent naturalness of herbs does not make them categorically "safe." Even herbs that are benign to most people have the potential for allergic reaction in some, and all herbal medicine treatment should be taken with knowledge and awareness of the potential dangers. Extra care should be taken by anyone who is elderly, very young, pregnant, immunocompromised, or in a weakened state.

Traditionally, herbal medicine would be administered by a doctor who would remain in close contact with the patient, and who could make adjustments to the treatment as needed. Statements such as "This herb is good for you," with the "you" being the generic population, are rare in TTM. The "you" in this sentence refers to a specific person with a specific Elemental imbalance. Many herbs may treat a condition; however, every herb is not right for every person. We implore you to use this book for informational purposes only, until you have adequate training and knowledge to evaluate your patients on an individual basis.

Contents

Appendix

C. Pierce Salguero

When I initially compiled the information that would become the first edition of this book in the late 1990s, I was in my early twenties, living in Chiang Mai and just beginning to study many different aspects of Thai healing. Information in English on Traditional Thai Medicine was hard to come by in those days, and I had the vision to write a series of books to make what I was learning—while I was learning it—available to a general public that had little awareness of Thai traditions. The notes I was taking on Thai herbal medicine became the first volume in a series with Findhorn Press, which went on to include books on massage and spiritual healing traditions as well. Now, returning to these books after over 15 years of academic study of Asian medical traditions, I see clearly the enthusiasm of youth and the excitement of discovery on every page, and I remember those times in Chiang Mai fondly.

There is a timeless myth in traditional medical circles that "true" or "authentic" knowledge is to be found only in the earliest, most original text, and that later versions are corrupt, debased, or untrustworthy. In scholarly circles, however, we know the opposite to be true. We know that our collective scholarship deepens from generation to generation, that individual scholars become better informed over a lifetime study, and that any edition of a book—but especially a first edition—is always a snapshot of a work in progress.

While the second edition of this book is as much a work in progress as the first, it has improved considerably upon the previous version—so much so that, in my opinion, it should be considered a completely new book. The first edition was compiled from bits and pieces of information I was taught on an ad hoc basis by a wide range of herbalists, massage therapists, market sellers, and neighbors, as well as things I read in the books I had access to, on websites, and in tourist magazines. The second edition is informed by much deeper formal study. It has corrected a number of errors, misperceptions, and mistranslations in the first, and has included many other improvements, large and small. Where the first edition had no awareness of Thai medical history, this one does. Where the first introduced a single Taste system, this one introduces five. Where the first drew upon parallels and examples from Chinese, Indian, and Western herbal medicine, this one is confident enough to allow Thai medicine to stand on its own terms. The second edition also includes Thai script, Thai language resources in the bibliography, and includes an English translation of a Traditional Thai Medicine text.

If, indeed, this edition marks a great leap forward in the quality of the information on Thai medicine available in English, and if it improves so substantially upon the first, this is due only in small part to my own deepening knowledge. The majority of the credit must be given to my collaborators, Nephyr and Tracy. While in the years since the 1990s I have left behind my studies of Thai medicine in favor of becoming a scholar of medical history, Nephyr has been diligently studying herbal medicine with a wide range of Thai practitioners. She has also accumulated a great amount of experience teaching these traditions herself, and so she brings to this book both her practical experience with the herbs as well as her natural, laid-back way of explaining how to use them. Tracy, on the other hand, is a translator who initially became interested in learning the language after studying Thai massage. She has recently begun to turn her attention to the arcane and difficult language of historical medical texts and has now completed the first English translation of a Thai medical text since the 1970s. I think you will agree that the contributions both Nephyr and Tracy are making to the community of Thai massage and medicine practitioners through their writings and translations are something for which we should all be grateful.

I was very thankful that Nephyr and Tracy agreed to come on board to update and improve this book, and have enjoyed working with them greatly. Our process involved a lot of conversations back and forth between the three of us or in pairs, and I have a learned a lot myself from these exchanges. I have taken a backseat in the production of the second edition—acting more like an editor or project manager than an author—and consider this very much to be their book. Though I have, of course, read the book numerous times over the past few months, I have not yet tried many of the formulas and recipes Nephyr has recommended here, and I look forward to experimenting with them along with you, the reader. As we continue to learn together, my wish for us is that we may continue to approach Thai healing traditions with the spirit of enthusiasm and excitement of discovery that comes naturally to a new student. And that we continue to be open to growth and change, recognizing that wherever we are in our studies there is always the possibility of a lifetime of further learning.

Dr. C. Pierce Salguero
Durham, North Carolina
September 9, 2013

Nephyr Jacobsen

There is a room at The Naga Center, my little Thai massage and medicine school in Portland Oregon, that I love above most other rooms. It is dark and a bit hidden—a branch off the attic. It is where magic begins. The walls are lined with shelves, and the shelves are home to jar upon jar of dried herbs. And under one of the shelves, there sit gallons of concoctions, oils, and alcohols busy extracting the vital medicinal essence of the chopped and ground herbs that they are thick with. Some of these tinctures take as long as six months before they are ready for use, and I like to visit them as they quietly come into being.

There is something about plant medicine that takes me out of the business of my life and grounds me in the earthy solidity of roots and bark and leaves, bits of the gardens and forests that have been gathered together for the purpose of helping, of easing suffering, and of healing the hurts. It finds its way into my classes, into my healing arts practice, and into my kitchen, where I incorporate Thai medicine concepts into the dance of preparing food for family and friends.

I started out as a bodyworker, 20-plus years ago. The journey in massage therapy led to me to Thailand in the mid-1990s, where I began my study of Thai physical therapies, and soon I became a regular in the journey to the other side of the world. Now, as I write this preface, I am halfway through a two-year stay in Thailand, living in the mountains of the far north where the roots of traditional Thai medicine still flourish. A 15-minute walk through town takes me past four different market shops and stands selling medicinal herbs and formulas. The prevalence of nearby Hill Tribe villages and northern Thailand Lanna culture means that I regularly meet people who, upon learning that I am interested in traditional medicine, tell me "my mother knows herbs," or "my aunt grows medicine herbs," or "I know a man who gathers wild honey for the herbalists." Life here is saturated with Thai herbal medicine.

The use of herbs crept into my Thai massage practice through Thai balms that ease aching muscles, hot herbal compresses that perform miracles on pain-filled bodies, and eventually liniments that assist in healing acute injuries. The efficacy of these products has changed dramatically and forever my relationship with bodywork, as I have seen healing results that were never possible through physical manipulation alone. And as the external application of herbs became integral to the Thai physical therapies I practice and teach, knowledge of the internal use of herbs through food and medicine grew. When illness visited my own circles, I began more and more to reach for a Thai herbal capsule, or to get out the mortar and pestle and start mixing and mashing. As my understanding of Thai Element theory grew, it changed my approach to cooking as well. I started to think about the season and the individual health state of those I cook for, looking at all food as internal medicine. As a result, my family has never been more healthy.

When Pierce Salguero, the first person to teach me about the history of Thai medicine, asked me to participate in the revision of *A Thai Herbal*, I was honored and thrilled at the chance to share with others the things I have been learning. I was also humbled, for I am, and will likely always be, a novice in the world of Thai herbal medicine. Working on this project has taken a great deal of research, and a great deal of help. It simply could not have been done without the guidance of Tevijjo Yogi. For his willingness to spend hours translating old texts, answering my endless questions, pouring over lists of herbs and tastes with me, I give thanks. To Erin Wright, who has been holding down the fort at The Naga Center while I tromp around Thailand writing books, I give thanks. To Sunhaporn Keeratiadisal (Jeab), my glorious Thai language teacher and friend (you didn't even know how much your teaching was helping me sort out herb names), I give thanks. To Aaron and Django, my sweet husband and son, who have been abandoned for weeks at a time while I worked on this, I give thanks. To Pierce, for welcoming me into the unraveling and re-weaving of his book, I give thanks. And in Thai tradition, I give thanks to my parents, Mark, Gaby, and Star, for being my first teachers.

To the readers of this herbal: This book alone will not make you an herbalist. Learning traditional healing arts takes time and requires a teacher. But if we can bring you a sampling, if we can offer you a peek through the door, if we can show a little bit about the beauty and complexity and the joy of Thai herbal medicine, then for that, I give thanks. By the time this is published, I expect I'll be living once again in Portland, Oregon—once again finding comfort in my little herb room in the attic of The Naga Center. I'll have brought back with me many more roots and seeds and dried leaves to fill the room with the smells and energies of Thailand. And I'll happily gather with my students and friends to turn those herbs into balms and liniments and compresses, as together we make magic.

Nephyr Jacobsen
Chiang Rai, Thailand
August 12, 2013

How to Use This Book

There are many different ways that this book may be approached. If you are a trained herbal medicine practitioner, it will be a rough manual, an herbal reference compendium, perhaps an inspiration to try new things. If you are a Thai bodywork practitioner, then this book introduces you to practices that can support Thai bodywork, such as incorporating hot herbal compresses, heating balms, and liniments into a massage practice. If you are a novice herbalist, someone who likes the do-it-yourself approach to life, it will offer you simple formulas for household herbal products, treatments for mild conditions such as lice and the common cold, and the contents of a Thai herbal first-aid kit. For those with a love of the kitchen, it presents Thai cooking as a delicious way to maintain health, with an understanding of how what we eat affects our internal balance. And for those interested in history and culture, it provides a glimpse into ancient traditions still being practiced in one corner of the world.

Regardless of which sort of reader you are (and indeed you may be more than one), here are a few bits and pieces of guidance to help you to wade through:

- Before you dive straight into the recipes or formulas, we encourage you to read about the Elements, as this will bring greater understanding of the system as a whole before you get into its specifics.

- In this book, as is typical in discussions of herbal medicine, the word "herb" may apply to any substance ingested or absorbed into the body though skin, inhalation, eyes, or suppositories. This includes plants, animals, clay, stones, insects, and antlers.

- Measurements, whether they are for culinary recipes, household products, compresses and balms, or teas and pills, are rarely exact. When it comes to culinary recipes we encourage you to play. Taste, add more of this; taste, add more of that. Herbal compresses also have lots of room for experimenting. With herbal medicines such as balms and internal formulas, you should stick more closely to the formula, but even here it is usually okay if you have slightly more or less of something than asked for. In fact, this is how one can use the recipes given here as a basis for customizing individualized treatments.

- When making Thai medicinal formulas, it's best to use earthenware containers and to mix the herbs in a clay bowl or pot. Glass or ceramic containers are also acceptable. Stainless steel is okay, too, although it is not preferable. Aluminum and plastics are considered toxic and should not be used for medicine or food.

- Traditional Thai medicine is never neat and tidy, and often it is quite messy. In researching and writing this book, we have gathered information from a combination of historical texts, modern papers, and direct transmission from teachers—but regardless of the sources, we have stuck to presenting information as it was recorded and taught to us. Thus, the information for individual herbs presented in one part of the book sometimes strays outside of the codified lists that are presented elsewhere.

  For example, "chum" is a Thai word used to describe a strong, musky, odiferous taste that is often considered unpleasant, such as associated with the resinous rhizome asafoetida or the fruit durian. (In the West, this word could describe truffle oil or certain extra-ripe cheeses.) This word, which appears from time to time in the compendium, is not to be found in the Taste chapters. Since we are passing knowledge along and not inventing it, we ask our readers to roll with these inconsistencies, as we ourselves have learned to do.

- In the back of this book there is a translation of a traditional Thai medical text, the *Wetchasueksa Phaetsatsangkhep*, translated by Tracy Wells. The perceptive reader will likely spot some subtle differences between this translation and the information presented in the main text of this book. Most of these differences are simply matters of wording. While Tracy's goal was to provide an accurate translation, our job in the rest of the book was to present the teachings in a way that could be best understood by a newcomer to Thai medicine. Some of the differences, on the other hand, are the result of the fact that different texts and teachers in Thailand do not always match up perfectly. Since none of the differences are dramatic and the basic teaching is consistent, we have left them as they are.

CHAPTER 1

Introduction to Traditional Thai Medicine

History of Medicine in Thailand

Known as the Kingdom of Siam until 1939, and thereafter as the Kingdom of Thailand, for simplicity, in this book we refer to the region as "Thailand," regardless of which era we are discussing. Although historical records of the practice of medicine in Thailand begin only in the Ayutthaya period (1351–1767), common belief says that traditional Thai medicine preserves knowledge that has been handed down orally for over two thousand years by lineages of teachers and students. The ancient history of Thai medicine remains beyond the ability of historians to reconstruct conclusively. However, it is likely that at least some of the herbal knowledge that is still practiced in Thailand today has indeed been in existence for millennia, given that people have inhabited Southeast Asia for an estimated 1–2 million years and that people have always reached out to the natural world to heal their ailments and improve their health.

Much speculation exists about the primary influencing factors in the historical development of Thai medicine, and we will discuss these below. However, it must be noted that, despite the influx of knowledge from multiple cultures, traditional medicine always develops in close relationship with the geographical region in which it is practiced. The reason for this is that climate, soil, water, flora, and fauna affect the nature of diseases and injuries existent in any given region, as well as the natural medicinal options available. Hence, regardless of the many cultural influences that have gone into the tradition, Thai medicine can be said to be a product of the geographical region currently known as Thailand.

Thailand is bordered to the west by Burma, which exposed the territory to many influences from the Mon culture; to the east by Cambodia, bringing Khmer influence; and to the north by Laos and China, allowing exchange of ideas with these groups as well. Mon and Khmer peoples inhabited the land that is now Thailand long before the arrival of the Tai/Dai peoples, the ethnic group that today makes up the majority population in Thailand. Influences from these neighboring peoples continue to be reflected in many aspects of Thai culture. They are the source of many of Thailand's traditions of spirit-religion and folk belief, and, following the Indianization of Burma and Cambodia, the route by which Indian theories and beliefs entered Thailand as well. The modern nation of Thailand is also home to a wide range of people that have been given the umbrella term "Hill Tribes." The Hill Tribes living in Thailand represent a variety of separate ethnic groups with ancestral homelands in Tibet, China, and all over Southeast Asia. The migrations of the Tai peoples into the area about AD 800–1000, primarily from southern China via northern Vietnam, marked the beginning of a change in the dominant ethnic demographics. The Tais brought their own indigenous knowledge and beliefs into the mix of medical doctrines prevalent in the area.

Local legends attribute much of traditional Thai medicine to the ancient *reusi* (a Thai word derived from the Sanskrit *ṛṣi* or *rishi*), who are revered ascetics and seers. Known to study the natural sciences, such as astronomy, mathematics, and medicine, the reusi are credited with introducing many traditional herbal formulas, as well as with creating a system of self-care known as *reusi da ton*. Reusi da ton includes meditation, self-massage, range-of-motion exercises for the joints, and yoga-like postures. It has aspects that are similar to Indian yoga, and is one of the ingredients in the genesis of Thai massage.

While the reusi are said to have contributed specific herbal lore, medical techniques, and bodywork, the primary figurehead in traditional Thai medicine is the Buddha. As Thailand is 95–98 percent Buddhist, a substantial portion of the population considers the Buddha to be the ultimate physician and Buddhism to be the ultimate source of healing. Another Buddhist figure that is important is Jīvaka Komārabacha (known colloquially as "Jīvaka," "Shivago," or "Mor Chewok" หมอชีวก). Jīvaka is a doctor whose story is recorded in the sacred Buddhist text called the Vinaya, which is written in the ancient Pāli language. In this text, he is said to have been the physician to the Buddha and the original order of monks, and he therefore holds a role of great prominence in Thailand. In the north of the country, he is commonly called the "Father Doctor" (*pôrmŏr* พ่อหมอ). Many Thais embellish the stories about Jīvaka from the Buddhist scripture, saying that he traveled to Thailand and directly contributed medical knowledge to the area's healers. Today, medical practitioners in Thailand, from herbalists, dentists and midwives to biomedical surgeons, give homage to Doctor Jīvaka as a part of daily life. However, strictly speaking, there is no historical record of him traveling to Thailand, or even that he was a real person.

Aside from the legends of Jīvaka, many other Indian medical doctrines, stories, and lore arrived in Thailand in several waves throughout the first millennium AD. Thailand sits at the crossroads of an extensive trade network, and a constant flow of new information came into Thailand as Indian, Chinese, and Arab merchants plied their trade in the region. European explorers arrived as early as 1504. Thai medical traditions picked up something from each of these groups as they came through. With a length of 1,648 kilometers and a width of 780 kilometers, Thailand encompasses many different terrains, and different cultural groupings. At the bottom of the isthmus one finds Malay and Muslim people, while central Thailand has a strong Chinese population. In Northern Thailand, the "Lanna region" preserves many indigenous traditions of the Tai as well as Hill Tribe peoples.

As a result of this diverse mix of peoples and cultures, traditional Thai medicine varies significantly from practitioner to practitioner. Depending on heritage, training, and geographical location within Thailand, one person may incorporate more Chinese practices, another more Indian theory, and another more indigenous ideas. By about 1600, however, Thai temples and hospitals under royal patronage began codifying a system of medical theory and practice. What some scholars have called the "royal tradition" was based on the same ideas as the rural medical lore but became organized and systematized with an overlay of Ayurvedic and Western concepts. In 1836, King Rama III ordered an extensive renovation of the grounds of Wat Phra Chettuphon Wimon Mangklaram (commonly referred to as "Wat Pho" or "Wat Po"), which had been established as the royal temple in the new capital of Bangkok in the late 1700s. At that time, 60 inscribed stone tablets bearing Thai acupressure charts and 1,100 herbal recipes were placed in the walls of a temple to preserve medical knowledge for future generations. Over 80 statues depicting massage techniques and reusi da ton postures were erected throughout the grounds as well. These statues and stone tablets can still be seen by visitors to the temple today.

From 1895 to 1907, Wat Pho's traditional medical school published several important herbal manuals to disseminate the information collected at the temple throughout Thailand. These represent the main sources of historical information about medical practice in Thailand and are often cited as the definitive word on traditional Thai medicine. But it is important to remember that the codification of medicine sponsored by kings and preserved at Wat Pho represents a relatively small sample of the vast scope of traditional medicine in Thailand. Tellingly, a small handful of older texts have been preserved from the Bangkok and Ayutthaya periods (one famous example is the medical manuscripts of King Narai), and these frequently have little to do with the medical systematization at Wat Pho. Traditional doctors throughout Thailand to this day still keep hand-written notes and manuscripts handed down through generations, but these are fiercely guarded and not likely to become publicly available any time soon. Thus, it is perhaps inevitable that the true history of medicine in Thailand will always be more diverse and complex than the existing written sources lead us to believe.

Traditional Medicine Today

Today, multiple systems of traditional medicine coexist in Thailand. Below, we have mentioned four major and widely recognized traditions:

- **TRADITIONAL THAI MEDICINE (TTM)** (*Pâet păen tai* แพทย์แผนไทย)
  The standardized system promoted by the Ministry of Public Health and taught in colleges all over Thailand. It is based on certain ancient texts, was first standardized during the reign of the Fifth King in the late 19th century, and has been modified as recently as the late 1990s. This system is primarily derived from royal traditions of medicine, with considerable Western influence.

- **TRADITIONAL MEDICINE OF THAILAND** (*Pâet păen boh-raan* แพทย์แผนโบราณ)
  Non-standardized practices that are based on ancient texts written in Thai and Khmer script from the 19th century and before. Methods vary from practitioner to practitioner, depending on which texts they follow. *Mŏr păen boh-raan* translates to "traditional doctor."

- **LOCAL MEDICINE OR INDIGENOUS MEDICINE** (*Pâet péun bâan* แพทย์พื้นบ้าน)
  Local practices that vary from area to area and are based on local texts and teachings. Also known as "village medicine" (*Mŏr péun bâan* translates to "village doctor").

- **LANNA MEDICINE** (*Pâet láan-naa* แพทย์ล้านนา)
  Peoples of northern Thailand consider themselves to be Lanna, culturally distinct from Thais in other parts of the country. Lanna medicine is based on northern texts written in the Lanna script, and is a particularly well preserved tradition of local medicine. *Mŏr láan-naa* translates to "Lanna doctor." While in one sense, Lanna medicine is a specific local tradition of medicine, it is also an important source of knowledge for TTM. As Chiang Mai has emerged as an important center for health-related tourism in recent decades, Lanna medicine has been particularly influential in recent years, both among Western tourists and Thais themselves.

All of the above systems have mutually influenced one another, and they subsequently share many theories and practices. In practice, herbalists do not necessarily stick to only one category, but instead draw from multiple systems in their treatment of patients. While the compendium of herbs and formulas included in this book incorporates teachings from all four systems, the theoretical systems of Elements and Flavors introduced here are TTM.

There are five primary branches of TTM, with further specialization possible within each branch. The five primary branches are as follows (with an explanation of the literal meaning of the Thai name):

- **INTERNAL/HERBAL MEDICINE** (*Pâet-sàat* แพทยศาสตร์)
  Pâet = medicine, doctor, drugs
  Sàat = knowledge, study, science
  This branch includes the methods of using plants, animals, and minerals as medicine for both internal and external application, the use of food as medicine, dietary counseling, and the administration of medicine.

- **EXTERNAL THERAPIES OR ORTHOPEDIC MEDICINE** (*Gaai-yá-pâap bam-bàt* กายภาพบำบัด)
  Gaai-yá-pâap = body
  Bam-bàt = therapy
  This branch includes Thai massage. However, it is inclusive of many more therapies, including bone-setting, cupping, scraping, blood letting, point therapy, *sên* เส้น (channel) therapy, and much more.

- **DIVINATION OR ORACULAR SCIENCES** (*Hŏh-raa-sàat* โหราศาสตร์)
  Hŏh-raa = an astrological chart
  Sàat = knowledge, study, science
  This branch primarily uses Vedic astrology in order to ascertain a patient's Elemental constitution, disease predisposition, current illnesses, planetary influence, and remedial measures for afflictions caused by the planets. Palm reading, numerology, tarot, geomancy, and various other methods can also be employed in this branch of medicine.

- **SPIRIT MEDICINE** (*Săi-yá-sàat* ไสยศาสตร์)
  Săi-yá = magic
  Sàat = knowledge, study, science
  This branch of TTM involves demons, deities, and ghosts, and employs the use of invocations, mantras, amulets, and spiritual tattooing. A wide range of practices fall under this umbrella, which are often collectively referred to as "animism" or "shamanism."

- **BUDDHISM** (*Pút-tá-sàat* พุทธศาสตร์)
  Pút-tá = the Thai pronunciation of the word Buddha
  Sàat = knowledge, study, science
  Buddhist wisdom, practices, and beliefs are central to virtually all forms of traditional medicine in Thailand, and can be seen even in the most secular institutions of TTM. Buddhism is thought of as a system to alleviate all suffering, but this branch of medicine might be thought of as traditional Thai psychology as it is used predominantly to promote mental health and treat mental disorders.

Note that while TTM is officially divided into these five branches, there is also one more, less frequently mentioned branch: midwifery (*pà-dung kan* ผดุงครรภ์). Most likely, this branch is often forgotten because it is highly specialized and only practiced by women.

Practitioners of TTM rarely practice all five branches, but rather specialize in one branch, or perhaps even one aspect of one branch. At the same time, they know enough about all of the other branches to augment their speciality and create a holistic practice. It is frequently said that Thai medicine is a system that cares for body (internal and external medicine branches), mind (Buddhism branch), and spirit (divinatory and spirit medicine branches), making for a complete system that treats the whole being. All of these branches of TTM are bound together by Thai Element theory and Buddhist perspectives (which, while it is its own branch, is integral to all branches). As Thai Element theory is the foundation for all TTM, it will be discussed more in depth later in this book.

Traditional Thai Medicine
in the Future

For centuries, traditional medicine in Thailand has been an organically evolving system, which to a certain degree it remains today. However, governmental efforts to preserve and codify medical knowledge has had the effect of discouraging many of the local variations, and has introduced a stronger preference for Indian and Western concepts than previously existed. Today, one must put in extra effort to find practitioners outside of the government standardization regime who remain true to older Thai traditions. This standardization of Thai medicine is a double-edged sword. On the one hand, it brings a certain level of consistency to the practice of medicine and helps in the preservation of knowledge; on the other, it means that knowledge not approved by the government is in danger of being lost.

Since the early 1900s, Western scientific medicine has been making its mark on TTM. Today, while Thailand has many state-of-the-art biomedical hospitals that cater to the medical tourism demands of a global patient clientele, most modern urban and rural Thais continue to utilize the arts of massage, herbal healing, and spiritual healing in addition to modern medical technology from the West. The government of Thailand, in fact, is one of the biggest supporters of this blend of traditional and modern healing. In rural areas that remain far from Western-style hospitals, government-operated herbal clinics dispense traditional remedies alongside biomedical drugs with the support and blessing of the World Health Organization and UNICEF. How these very different medical models interrelate and integrate is an ongoing challenge, and TTM practitioners argue that such attempts should begin with a holistic understanding of the human as not merely a physical entity but a complex interwoven system.

An additional factor currently affecting TTM is the relatively new interest in Thai massage coming from the West and Japan. Since the early 1980s, non-Thais have been traveling to Thailand in increasing numbers to learn this art form. The vast majority of these students speak little to no Thai and come for short amounts of time. The presence of these tourists has created an atmosphere in which hands-on techniques that are easily demonstrable without language fluency are prioritized, while the more complex concepts of traditional medical theory are deemphasized or omitted. Furthermore, as non-Thais return to their countries of origin, they write books and offer classes on Thai massage that tend to either offer no theory at all, or to overlay traditional Chinese medicine, Indian Ayurveda, or (most commonly) Indian hatha yoga theory on top of Thai techniques. The reason for this is that while there is a dearth of Western language information on Thai medicine theory, there is a plethora of information on Chinese and Indian medicine available. Eventually, Thai teachings that use Indian and Chinese theory circle back to Thailand as Western books get published there, and Westerners share with Thai people what they have learned. This cycle contributes to the loss of TTM concepts in educational settings in tourist areas across Thailand.

Thus, even as traditional medicine is experiencing a resurgence in Thailand, it is changing to meet the expectations of the government, the international medical community, and the local tourists. Today, traditional medicine in Thailand exists in many flavors: practitioners whose approach is based in ancient indigenous practices, practitioners who incorporate more Indian or Chinese ideas and techniques into a base of Thai medicine, a range of Hill Tribe healers, those who focus on the royal traditions, and those who employ the more recent standardized systems promoted by the government. Herbal medicine, in particular, reflects a wide variety of individual and local practices that depend on the region, climate, flora, local folklore, or particular village or family traditions. However, there also are many formulas for both internal and external herbal application that are commonly found throughout the land. In this book, we will remain focused on herbs, lore, and formulas that are commonly accepted as being truly "Thai"—whether from the official TTM system, the practices of the Lanna region, the royal traditions, or the teachings of our individual teachers— and will avoid wandering into Ayurvedic, Chinese, or Western practices.

CHAPTER 2

Thai Herbal Theory

The Elements

Thai Element theory has its roots in the Pāli Buddhist tradition. Like many other forms of traditional medicine in Europe and Asia, this tradition holds that all things are made of the Great Elements, and that it is the relative balance between these that is responsible for the variance of the universe. From urban asphalt to jungle leaves—even the character and the nature of our thoughts—everything is believed to be influenced by these basic Elements.

TTM holds that the body, too, is made up of Earth, Water, Fire, and Wind. (Though Thai healers primarily work with these Four Elements, they recognize a total of six: the standard four, plus Space and Consciousness.) While the underlying foundational system of TTM is similar to other traditions (such as Greek, Indian, and Arabic medicine), each culture has understood and explained the Elements in different ways. No one medical system can be simply substituted for another, and the Elements in Thai medicine must be understood within the Thai context.

The Elements refer not to physical substances but to qualities. For example, substances that are solid, hard, stable, and heavy can be said to have the qualities of the Earth Element. Substances that are cold, moist, fluid, and/or soft can be said to have the qualities of the Water Element. Knowing and understanding the attributes of each Element is vital to working with any aspect of TTM, and this is especially true in the case of herbal medicine.

Element	Experience	Function	Qualities	Temperature
Earth	Solidity	Provides resistance and support, like a skeleton, foundation, canyon wall, or building.	Hard Stable Heavy	Mild
Water	Liquidity	Provides cohesion and fluidity, like when drops of water merge.	Moist Fluid Soft	Cold
Fire	Heat	Provides transformation and ripening. Fire is the impetus for change.	Bright Reactive Sharp	Hot
Wind	Movement	Provides growth and vibration. Wind is responsible for all movement.	Light Rough Dry	Cool

According to the Four Element theory, the anatomy and physiology of the human body can be broken down into the following categories:

Element	Anatomy / Physiology	Within The Body
Earth	All that is solid, providing structure and containment	1. Hair on the head 2. Hair on the body 3. Nails 4. Teeth 5. Skin 6. Muscles 7. Sên ("channels," i.e., the tendons, ligaments, vessels, nerves) 8. Bones 9. Bone marrow 10. Kidneys 11. Heart 12. Liver/pancreas (in some TTM texts, these are considered one system) 13. Fascia (sometimes diaphragm, pleura) 14. Spleen 15. Lungs 16. Large intestine 17. Small intestine 18. Stomach (including recently eaten food and chyle) 19. Digested food and feces 20. Brain and central nervous system
Water	All bodily fluids, providing viscosity and cohesion	1. Bile 2. Phlegm in the respiratory tract 3. Pus and lymph 4. Blood 5. Sweat 6. Fat 7. Tears 8. Oil 9. Saliva 10. Mucus in the nose and throat 11. Synovial fluid 12. Urine
Fire	Warmth, digestion, breaking things down, motivation	1. Fire that causes aging and decay of the body 2. Fire that provides warmth to the body 3. Fire that digests 4. Fire that causes emotion and fever
Wind	All movement, from physical movement to the movement of thoughts	The Wind Element is conventionally divided into six types of Winds, as is similar to the teachings found in Buddhist texts: 1. Wind that moves from the top of the head to the feet/abdomen, depending on text (Descending Wind)

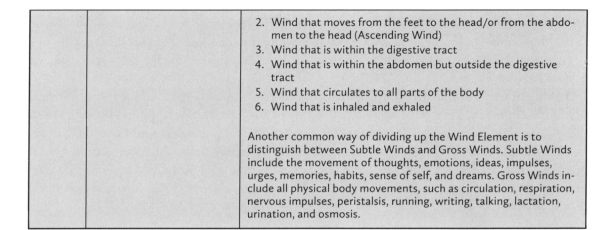

		2. Wind that moves from the feet to the head/or from the abdomen to the head (Ascending Wind) 3. Wind that is within the digestive tract 4. Wind that is within the abdomen but outside the digestive tract 5. Wind that circulates to all parts of the body 6. Wind that is inhaled and exhaled Another common way of dividing up the Wind Element is to distinguish between Subtle Winds and Gross Winds. Subtle Winds include the movement of thoughts, emotions, ideas, impulses, urges, memories, habits, sense of self, and dreams. Gross Winds include all physical body movements, such as circulation, respiration, nervous impulses, peristalsis, running, writing, talking, lactation, urination, and osmosis.

The constant interaction of the Four Elements gives rise to the processes of the human body, and is the impetus behind physical life. It is therefore of vital importance to do one's best to keep the Four Elements balanced. The Elements can become unbalanced due to a variety of reasons. Environmental factors can affect the body, for instance, when hot weather causes excitement of the Fire Element and weakening of the Water Element, or cold weather causes the Water Element to become amplified while weakening the Fire Element. Food can also affect the balance, as for instance when indulgence in spicy foods and alcohol causes excitement of the Fire Element, or indulgence in sweet and heavy foods causes excitement of the Water Element.

Elements can exist in various states, including:

- **BALANCED** (sà-má-dun สมดุล): A normal Element that is functioning in a manner that is healthy and balanced.

- **EXCITED** (*gam rêrp* กำเริบ): An excited Element is functioning at a more intense level than is healthy. Other terms that convey this state include "amplified," "intensified," and "agitated."

- **WEAKENED** (*yòn* หย่อน): A weakened Element is functioning with less vitality than is healthy. Another term that conveys this state is "depleted."

- **DISTORTED** (*pí-gaan* พิการ): A distorted Element is out of balance, or unstable, but not always clearly excited or weakened. It may fluctuate between the two.

- **BROKEN** (*dtaèk* แตก): A broken Element is a very serious condition, possibly but not necessarily fatal, that requires professional medical attention.

- **DISAPPEARED** (*hăi bpai* หายไป): Once any one Element is gone, the body is dying. We require all Elements to live.

While it is common for people to discuss the state of Elements in terms of "excessive" and "deficient," the quantity of the Element does not change within us; it is more apt to say that the vibrancy or the potency of the Element is prone to fluctuation. For this reason, we prefer to use terms such as "excited" and "weakened," or "amplified" and "subdued."

During the normal course of life, the balance of intensity of each Element fluctuates with age, season, environment, and diet. These fluctuations are natural and do not require moderation unless they sway too far from a healthy state, or occur outside of the expected parameters created by natural changes. It is important to take these factors into consideration before embarking on Elemental diagnosis. (For example, a slight increase in Wind excitement during the rainy season, when it is an expected fluctuation, is less likely to indicate a problem than an increase in Wind excitement during the hot season.)

Causes of Change in Elemental Balance

According to Four Element theory, there are three causes of a shift in the state of Elemental balance: natural, unnatural, and karmic. (The Earth Element, being the most stable, is often omitted in the following factors).

1. The Thirteen Natural Causes of Elemental Imbalance	
Elemental Fluctuations	Ongoing internal fluctuations of the Elements are natural. But, the relationship between the internal Elements is also affected by external factors, such as: **Wind:** Agitates the Wind Element within us. **Heat:** Agitates the Fire Element within us. **Dampness:** Agitates the Water Element within us. **Cold:** Can agitate Wind and Water within us. **Dryness:** Agitates Wind within us.
Season	**Hot Season:** Causes a natural excitement of the Fire Element. **Rainy Season:** Causes excitement of the Wind Element. (This point frequently causes confusion, as people associate rain with Water. However, in TTM, rain is associated with Wind because rainstorms involve lots of motion of wind and water, and motion is the quality of the Wind Element.) **Cold Season:** Causes excitement of the Water Element.
Time	**Wind** is more vibrant from 2–6 a.m. (or the 4 hours preceding sunrise), and again from 2–6 p.m. (or the 4 hours preceding sunset) **Water** is more vibrant from 6–10 a.m. (or the 4 hours post sunrise), and again from 6–10 p.m. (or the 4 hours post sunset) **Fire** is more vibrant from 10 a.m.–2 p.m. (or the two hours before and after the sun's zenith), and again from 10 p.m.–2 a.m. (or the two hours before and after midnight)
Age	**From birth to 8 years old:** Water Element is strong. (This is why children show Watery characteristics such as soft skin, large eyes, strong emotions, and a tendency toward mucusy diseases.)

Age cont.	**From 8–16 years old:** Water is waning, and Fire is waxing. (The emergence of Fire can be seen in an increase in acne, rebellion, and sexuality as the individual enters adolescence.) **From 16–32 years old:** Fire Element is strong (This is the peak of one's motivation, drive, and intellect.) **From 32–64 years old:** Fire is waning, while Wind is waxing. **From 64 years old until death:** Wind Element is strong and continues waxing. (This is seen in the tendencies of aged people to have dry fragile skin, smaller eyes, insomnia, constipation, arthritis, and anxiety.)
Region, Climate, Geography	The relative dryness, coldness, humidity, heat, and dampness of a geographical area all affect our Elemental balance. (For instance, living in a hot, dry climate will tend to agitate Fire and Wind, while living in damp cool climate will tend to agitate Water.) Likewise, the features of the geography also influence Elemental balance. An example of this would be living by a large body of still water (agitating Water Element) or living in a subterranean environment, such as a basement or cave (increased connection to Earth Element).
Daily Routine	How we go about our day affects the Elements. Inconsistent patterns in sleeping and eating erratically, for example, will lead to agitated Wind, as will constant stress and rushing about. Conversely, consistency and slow pacing may strengthen Water. Repeated bold actions and driven behavior may be signs of a Fire Element that is already strong, but may also assist in creating stronger Fire Element.
Eating	What we eat has a direct effect upon our Elemental balance. For instance, habitual intake of cold, moist foods, such as iced drinks and ice cream, will excite the Water Element and weaken the Fire Element. Diet is one of the primary factors in Elemental diagnosis and treatment.
Posture	Poor posture causes Elemental imbalance and has a particular effect on Earth and Wind Elements. For example, sitting hunched over for extended periods of time causes bound muscles (Earth) and constricts movement (Wind).
Sleep Patterns	Getting the right amount of sleep, at the right time, maintains Elemental balance. Sleeping too much or too little, or sleeping during the daytime, may lead to agitations of the Water Element.
Exercise and Work	The kind of exercise or work we engage in, the intensity with which we engage in it, and even the time of day in which we engage in it will affect our Elemental balance. (For example, hard exercise outside at midday will excite Fire, while an excessive amount of cardiovascular exercise agitates Wind.)
Extremes in Temperature	Temperature extremes cause Elemental imbalance. For example, those who live in hot climates but work in extremely cold, air-conditioned buildings are constantly shifting back and forth between hot and cold in a way that is unnatural and unsettles the Fire Element.
Natural Urges	Suppression of natural urges, such as belching, defecating, urinating, coughing, etc., causes Elemental imbalance.
Emotions	Indulgence in strong emotions (even excessive joy) will also cause Elemental imbalance. (For example, dwelling in anger will excite Fire, while anxiety excites Wind.)

While the previous chart included primarily environmental and behavioral factors, the next two lists include a number of factors that are part of the Thai religious and spiritual worldview.

2. The Six Unnatural Causes of Elemental Imbalance	
Ghosts/Spirits	Ghosts and spirits can cause various Elemental imbalances but most often affect Wind. (Traditionally, Thais have a strong belief in ghosts and spirits, collectively known as *pĕe* ผี.)
Deities	Any Element may be affected (positively or negatively) by deities. Thai religion recognizes a great number of deities from the Buddhist and Hindu pantheon.
Magic	Like deities, magical causes of Elemental imbalance may affect any Element. For example, if hexed with obesity, one is hexed with a Water problem.
Weapons	Weapons primarily affect Earth Element, as they break the skin, bones, organ structure, etc. This will, in turn, affect all other Elements.
Accidents	Most of the time, accidents will be the same as weapons, in that Earth Element is the first affected.
Poison	Poison can also affect any Element. It depends on the particular effect of the substance ingested, inhaled, or touched.

3. The Two Karmic Causes of Elemental Imbalance	
Past Karma	Past karma can predetermine one's Elemental makeup during in-utero development and is the result of choices made in previous lifetimes.
Present Karma	Present karma is determined by our actions and reactions in this lifetime.

Element Diagnostics

Diagnosing disease according to the Elements is a crucial part of Thai herbal medicine. Diagnostic skills take many years to develop, and traditionally Thai apprentices studied under able teachers for decades before they were considered to be healers in their own right. Some basic guidelines can be outlined. However, for serious conditions an experienced medical doctor must be sought out.

In the charts below, the Elements are listed in the order in which they become disturbed. Wind is generally the first Element to become imbalanced, due to it being the lightest and therefore the most easily blown off course. Earth, on the other hand, being the heaviest Element, is generally the last affected in the progression of a disease. Once it is affected, however, this usually means a serious condition. (For example, in a liver disease, imbalances of Fire and Wind would refer to problems with the *function* of the organ, but once Earth is involved we are talking about the *structure* of the liver itself being compromised. Also, conditions such as an abundance of tumors and other abnormal growths, as seen with serious cancers, are a result of Earth Element being affected.) An exception to the progression of the Elements is the event of sudden trauma that directly impacts Earth body parts—such as injury to the tissue, bones, tendons, and ligaments.

Examples of Elemental Imbalances - Excited State		
	Mental	**Physical**
Wind	Anxiety, insomnia, restlessness, attention deficit disorder. In cases of extreme imbalance, Tourette's Syndrome, obsessive-compulsive disorders, and insanity.	All symptoms of sharp pain, such as headaches, arthritis, and shooting pains. Conditions involving movement, such as restless leg syndrome, tics, hiccups, and other spasms. Constipation that results from excessive dryness, or diarrhea that results from too much downward Wind movement.
Fire	Tendency to anger and frustrate easily. Possibility of living "on overdrive," driven to succeed to the point of ill health.	Symptoms of redness, such as rash, acne, and boils. Problems with the liver and gallbladder, food digesting too quickly, and fever.
Water	Depression, lack of mental acuity, sadness	Lethargy, obesity, issues with reproductive and urinary systems. Mucus diseases, such as pneumonia, congestion, wet cough. Also, toxicity (Water is a heavy Element and tends to hold onto toxins).
Earth	Stubbornness, lack of mental acuity	Tumors, prolific growth of hair (especially in abnormal areas), bone spurs, extra bones and teeth, any overabundance of tissue.

Examples of Elemental Imbalances - Weakened State		
	Mental	**Physical**
Wind	Lack of mental acuity, lack of creativity and inspiration.	Any condition with impeded movement, such as paralysis, slow circulation, coma, frozen shoulder, food not moving through digestive system, certain types of constipation, or contracted muscles. Lethargy and exhaustion.
Fire	Lack of motivation, drive, mental acuity, sex drive, courage, or self-defense.	Poor digestion, lack of body heat, low blood pressure.
Water	Lack of mental cohesion, ungrounded characteristics.	Dryness in the lungs or intestines, thinness of blood, dry skin, reproductive issues, brittleness, lack of vitality, failure to thrive physically.
Earth	Signs of imbalance are similar to Water Element characteristics, such as lack of mental stability, ungrounded characteristics, flightiness, but are more ingrained and less malleable.	Weak, broken, or compromised bones, nails, hair, teeth, skin, organ structures, etc.

Five Sense Diagnosis

Traditionally, Thai medicine practitioners would use all five of their senses in making a diagnosis. They would use hearing to listen to their patient's complaints and needs. But, also to listen to how the patient speaks, their choice of words, their pacing and focus, as all these factors are clues to Elemental diagnosis. (For example, someone with overly excited Wind may speak quickly and have a hard time staying on topic.) Sight is used to examine the patient visually. The smell of a person's sweat, breath, and urine gives rise to vast amounts of information, including the ability to detect infection. Touch is used to palpate muscles, bones, tendons, and other tissues, to determine the quality of skin hydration and to take pulse readings. And, while it is not done as much in modern times, traditionally, the sense of taste was employed in tasting a patient's urine in order to gain further understanding of particular disease conditions. (In fact, the Thai name for what we call diabetes, translates to "Sweet urine disease." Since urine is sterile, this practice was not as dangerous as some might think.) While you may choose to skip the use of the sense of taste, it remains important to use as many senses as possible for a thorough examination of a condition.

Further Diagnostic Tools

Specific diagnostic tools employed in TTM are outlined below. Of course, they too employ the use of the practitioner's senses.

- **THAI PULSE DIAGNOSIS:** With Thai pulse diagnosis, the practitioner feels the patient's pulse, most often at the wrist, to determine Elemental balance and imbalance. It can take many years to become proficient at this diagnostic tool, but once mastered the practitioner can often determine exactly what is happening Elementally to each individual organ in the patient's body as well as the systemic state of the Elements.

- **THAI TONGUE DIAGNOSIS:** Tongue diagnosis in Thailand is used primarily to determine the state of the patient's digestive system but can also show some systemic conditions. The therapist looks at the shape, color, coating, and texture of the patient's tongue for diagnostic clues.

- **CUPPING AND SCRAPING:** These are techniques that have the unique quality of being both therapeutic and diagnostic. When the body is cupped or scraped, the resulting colors that appear on the skin can be used diagnostically.

- **OBSERVATION:** This is a very important diagnostic tool. Practitioners observe the patient's behavior, body, eyes, tongue, feces, urine, skin, nails, and more in order to learn causes and conditions of illness.

- **QUESTIONING:** In addition to the primary symptoms, a traditional medicine practitioner will generally want to know about the patient's diet, lifestyle, digestion, sleep patterns, menstrual cycles, work, elimination, and spiritual life. The more complete a picture the therapist can get, the more likely they can make an accurate diagnosis. Of special importance is diet. Knowing what the patient eats, how it is digested, and the condition of the resulting waste tells a TTM practitioner great quantities of information.

The tools above can be used to acquire very specific information about conditions and diseases, not only narrowing down what Element/s is/are out of balance, but even identifying individual body parts that are affected. (For instance, a practitioner might determine that a patient has overly excited Water in their lower digestive tract, or weakened mental Fire.) A more general diagnosis may be made by a newer practitioner by determining simply which Element is out of balance and then determining if it is excited, weakened, or distorted. When an Element is distorted it can be harder to diagnose. The symptoms will fluctuate between those of excitement and weakness, and there may be a sense of confusion and elusiveness in the diagnostic process. (For example, feeling the Wind pulse on someone with distorted Wind, one experiences the pulse speeding up, then slowing down, then disappearing and reappearing.) Broken and disappeared Elements are beyond the capacity of the ordinary practitioner to address and require professional emergency treatment.

The newcomer to Thai herbal medicine should keep in mind the above points, but should also recognize that diagnostic skill can sometimes be an art rather than a science (this is true even in modern scientific medicine). Symptoms can often manifest with a mix of excited and weakened states, and can appear in more than one organ system. (For example, a patient with excited Fire Element may also exhibit weakened Wind. This individual could manifest with heart disease, high blood pressure, high cholesterol, short temper, reddish color in the face, and a voracious appetite—all symptoms of Fire Element excitement. At the same time, he or she could exhibit lethargy, boredom, and sluggishness—all of which relate to Wind.)

Tastes

Once the affected Elemental imbalance has been pinpointed, and it has been determined whether the disease is a matter of excited, weakened, or distorted Elements, the Thai herbalist can prescribe dietary changes and herbal supplements to either strengthen or soothe this particular Element.

In traditional Thai herbal medicine, every ingestible substance is assigned a "Taste" classification. There are five different Taste systems found in TTM, named for the number of Tastes recognized in each:

1. The Nine Taste system is used when utilizing individual medicinal herbs internally.
2. The Eight Taste system is used when herbs are combined with a "vehicle," a substance that assists the body to absorb the medicine and direct it to the proper place.
3. The Six Taste system is used to understand herbs in everyday life, such as in foods.
4. The Four Taste system is used when herbs are applied externally.
5. The Three Taste system is used for herbal formulas that combine multiple herbs to be used medicinally internally.

The Six Taste system for everyday herbs will be elaborated upon in Chapter 3, and the Four Taste system for external herbs will be elaborated upon in Chapter 4. The others will be explained here.

Nine Taste System for Individual Herbs Used as Medicine

As mentioned above, the Nine Taste system is utilized when individual herbs are taken internally for medicinal purposes. (You will see that there are actually 10 categories listed here. This is still called the "Nine Taste System" because the 10th, "Tasteless," is not considered an actual Taste but the lack thereof.)

The information in the chart below can be used to determine which Taste category would be given to a patient to help with a given condition. It should be noted that combining multiple herbs for multiple conditions is not recommended, as not all herbs are compatible with one another and the combining itself may produce an entirely different effect.

Overview of the Nine Taste System		
Taste	**Therapeutic Use**	**Contraindications**
Astringent	Absorbs wetness, heals wounds, treats diarrhea and dysentery. Dries mucus and stools. Binds the Elements, hence is good for external wounds, stopping bleeding, cleansing and healing. *Binding*	Constipation, indigestion, distorted Fire Element, and diseases of Wind. Also contraindicated with presence of small, dry feces.
Sweet	Permeates and builds the tissue (making it abundant and healthy), treats general malaise, and provides strength. Also an energy tonic. *Permeating*	Mucus, diabetes, jaundice, lymph issues, and wounds.
Toxic	Treats poison and toxins in the body, including toxins arising from blood, and mucus. Treats poisonous animal and insect bites as well as parasites and skin conditions. Treats toxic fever. *Corrects poison*	Diseases of heart, bile, and cough.
Bitter	Lowers fever caused by blood or bile, increases appetite, helps with dehydration, treats blood problems, quenches excessive inner thirst. Bitter Taste is a tonic for the blood and bile. *Corrects blood*	Diseases of the heart. Diseases in which Wind causes pain (e.g., bloating, intestinal gas, etc.).

Spicy/Hot (This Taste has a sub-category of **Aromatic Pungent** herbs, which are not necessarily spicy but have a warming effect, such as cinnamon and cardamom.)	Treats diseases of Wind, flatulence, gas pain, indigestion, and chest and abdominal tightness. Moves blocked Wind, moves the Wind in the intestines, removes stagnant blood in the uterus, tonifies the Elements, treats distorted Elements, and moves menstrual blood. *Corrects Wind*	Diseases of Fire, high fevers, toxic fever (a traditional disease category that includes dangerous forms of fever and infectious diseases characterized by fever, such as dengue fever, scarlet fever, etc.).
Oily	Treats distortions in the *sên* (i.e., tendons, ligaments, nerves), lubricates joints, lubricates the body and allows smooth function of organs and tissue, supports the body heat, nourishes the bone marrow. Oily Taste is a tonic for tissue. *Corrects the sên*	Distortion of the Water Element, jaundice, cough, difficulty breathing, dysentery, and fevers.
Fragrant/Cool	Fragrant/Cool is a tonic for the heart-mind (in TTM, the heart is connected both to the physical organ and to mental/emotional well-being). Eases stress, anxiety, mental fog. Relieves stress of the fetus. Tonic for the liver and the lungs. This is the primary Taste for supporting the Subtle Winds. *Refreshing*	Diseases of the Gross Winds, gas pain, other pain in the body caused by Wind.
Salty	Permeates the skin and the mucus membrane, treats some skin diseases, preserves tissue (prevents putrefaction), removes mucus from the colon, and is beneficial for conditions with dry small feces. *Permeates the skin*	Diseases that cause problems with elimination, diarrhea, internal bleeding, dysentery.
Sour	Treats diseases of mucus and cough, cleanses the blood, expels toxins, and is a purgative. *Cuts mucus*	Problems of the lymph, wounds, loose stools, toxic fever, and diarrhea.
Tasteless	Calms diseases of Fire, acts as a diuretic, decreases mucus, treats mild fever, relieves dehydration and inner heat, helps support kidneys, treats fever and some kinds of toxic fever, absorbs poison, relieves dehydration and thirst. *Corrects Mucus*	Low blood pressure.

Examples of the Nine Tastes from Traditional Thai Texts		
Astringent	**Sweet**	**Toxic**
Tea leaves Pomegranate rind Mangosteen rind Tamarind leaves Betel nut Unripe banana	Safflower flowers Licorice root Annatto flower Sugar cane Palm fruit Milk Honey	Marijuana Nux vomica Candelabra bush Opium Pomegranate root Datura Python bones Sulphur Arsenic
Bitter	**Spicy/Hot**	**Oily**
Guduchi Andrographis Neem Bitter melon Gall bladder of various animals	Garlic Basil Camphor Clove Ginger Plumbago Long pepper Asafoetida Mace Black pepper	Sesame seeds Water chestnut Many beans & nuts Lotus seed Coconut meat Various animal milks (especially goat milk) Various animal livers Egg yolk Costus root Mung bean Cashew Lotus root Sichuan lovage root
Fragrant/Cool	**Salty**	**Sour**
Ylang ylang Heartwood of white and red sandalwood Saffron Rose Chrysanthemum Jasmine Lotus stamens Myrrh	Onion leaf Salt Potassium nitrate Seafood Seaweed Potassium chloride Cuttlefish bone Oyster shell	Roselle Kaffir lime fruit Lime fruit Senna leaf Starfruit Sorrel Alum
Tasteless		
Pine wood Clay Morning glory Lime tree root		

Eight Taste System

The Eight Taste system relates to how tastes permeate to different parts of the body and is used primarily when herbs are combined with a *vehicle*. A vehicle is a substance that supports the herb by directing it to the right place (e.g., alcohol transports medicinal effects to the *sên*), or by boosting the herb's effectiveness. The Eight Taste system uses the same tastes as the Nine Taste system, but with the omission of Toxic and Tasteless.

Bitter	Permeates to the skin
Astringent	Permeates to the tissue (muscle, fascia, fat)
Salty	Permeates to the *sên* (tendons, ligaments, nerves, circulatory vessels)
Spicy/Hot	Permeates to the bone
Sweet	Permeates to the large intestine
Sour	Permeates to the small intestine
Fragrant/Cool	Permeates to the heart
Oily	Permeates to the joints throughout the body

Three Taste System for Compound Medicinal Formulas

Once multiple herbs are combined into a medicinal formula, the Three Taste system is employed. Formulas will have either a warming, cooling, or neutral effect.

Three Tastes of Medicinal Compound Formulas			
Heating	Treats the Gross Winds (some say treats Water)	Expels blood, nourishes the Elements, creates movement. Used during the rainy season to calm Wind.	Contraindicated in cases of toxic fever.
Cooling	Treats Fire Element	Treats toxic fever, subdues poison. Used during the hot season.	Contraindicated in diseases of Wind.
Mild (neither heating nor cooling)	Treats Water Element (some say treats Wind)	Treats the Subtle Winds, treats mucus and blood. Used during the cold season.	Contraindicated in toxic fevers.

How the Tastes Affect the Elements

All ingested substances exert their medicinal effects on the body through the effects of the Tastes on the Elements. Each of the 13 Taste categories introduced above has a specific effect on the Elements. While TTM texts do not elaborate on exactly how each of these tastes treats each Element in all cases, in practice we can observe the following:

Treats Earth	Treats Water	Treats Wind	Treats Fire
Astringent	Sour	Mild	Cool
Sweet	Bitter	Spicy/Hot	Heating
Oily	Toxic		Fragrant/Cool
Salty			Tasteless

EARTH: Astringent binds and firms the Earth Element. Sweet nourishes or builds the Earth Element (specifically the tissue). Oily supports Earth by keeping it lubricated and functioning smoothly, and Salty preserves it.

WATER: Sour purifies and liquifies the Water Element. Bitter is nourishing to the blood and the bile, and Toxic treats diseases of Water and poison (in all Elements, but especially in the Water Element).

WIND: Mild balances the Subtle Winds, and calms and supports the smooth function of Wind. Spicy/Hot treats the Gross Winds and causes the movement of the Winds. It also purges Wind.

FIRE: Cool and Fragrant/Cool diminish Fire, while Heating increases it. Tasteless treats fever and toxicity, reducing Fire and inflammation.

CHAPTER 3

Everyday Herbs

Food Therapy, or Everyday Medicine

According to a legend told in Buddhist scripture, when the "Father Doctor" Jīvaka was a young man, he was given his final examination by his master. He was challenged to go off into the forest and find a plant that could not be used as a medicine. After searching a large area, Jīvaka returned and declared to his teacher that everything he saw was, in fact, medicinal. At that point the master knew that Jīvaka had completed his training. It is with this philosophy that traditional healers have approached the world for thousands of years, and it is this philosophy that continues to form the backbone of traditional Thai medicine.

Because of the connections between the sense of taste and the medicinal effects on the body, everything we put in our mouths (even things that are tasteless) transforms our bodies and minds. Many medicinal herbs mentioned throughout this collection are ingested every day in the typical Thai diet. In traditional Thai cuisine, almost every dish is considered to be therapeutic in some way or another. In fact, the Thai herbalist traditionally will recommend modifications to the diet before recommending more powerful herbal medicines. An old Thai proverb says that all diseases originate in the food we eat. In the West, we also say "we are what we eat." If we eat well, we will enjoy health, well-being, and longevity; if we eat poorly, we will become unhealthy, unhappy, and prone to illness.

The Six Tastes System

As mentioned in Chapter 2, one of the Taste classification systems in Thailand uses six flavor categories to explain the medicinal effects of food. It is important to understand that this is a completely different system than the Nine Taste system. For example, many foods that fall into the Oily Taste in the Nine Taste system in fact fall into the Sweet Taste category in the Six Taste system. This latter system is used when approaching the foods that we eat for nourishment, with the goal of eating for optimal health.

Six Tastes Used in Food			
Taste	Amplifies	Subdues	Temperature
Bitter	Wind	Water and Fire	Cooling
Spicy/Hot	Wind and Fire	Water	Warming
Astringent	Wind	Fire and Water	Cooling

Salty	Water and Fire	Wind	Warming
Sour	Water and Fire	Wind	Warming
Sweet	Water	Wind and Fire	Cooling

Ideally, a balanced meal will include all Six Tastes. Individual dishes have particular flavor profiles and should be combined with intention. (For example, Thai tom yum soup contains all Six Tastes, however it is weighted toward the Spicy/Hot, and is therefore balancing for Wind and Water. Eating sweet mango with sticky rice may be beneficial for someone whose Wind is amplified, while it is less so to one with amplified Water Element.) By combining the right flavors in the right combinations, a meal can balance the Elements and support the health needs of the eater.

While it is best to base these decisions on the individual who will consume the meal, one can also use seasons to aid in the choice. Perhaps the easiest way to get started with this approach to cooking is to simply decide if you wish for the meal to be cooling or warming. Cooling meals should be taken in hotter weather, and warming meals in colder weather in order to counteract the effects of the climate. If you wish it to be cooling, look for flavors that will subdue the Fire Element. If you wish it to be warming, look for those that amplify the Fire Element.

Examples of Foods Classified by Six Tastes

Taste	Example
Bitter	Bitter greens (arugula, kale, collards, dandelion), lime rind, radicchio
Spicy/Hot	Black pepper, chilies, garlic. (Aromatic Pungents include cinnamon, nutmeg, cardamom, ginger)
Astringent	Unripe bananas, tea leaves, pomegranate skin, turmeric
Salty	Celery, seaweed, fish, seafood, salt
Sour	Lemons, limes, vinegar, yogurt, starfruit
Sweet	Licorice, watermelon, coconut, dates, mango, sugar, honey, milk

In addition to taking Tastes into account, a knowledge of the health properties of individual ingredients is useful. Knowing that, say, nutmeg is good for the heart, or that licorice is good for the lungs, will go a long way toward creating meals that bring health to those who eat them. See Chapter 6 for more about the benefits of specific herbs.

Avoiding Toxins

In our opinion, Jīvaka's motto that everything is medicine should be reinterpreted in modern times. Certain man-made foods that are available today are so toxic to the system that we would argue they don't have enough redeeming nutritional or medicinal qualities to offset the dangers of eating them. Herbalists, natural healers, and traditional nutritionists the world over have warned that the following modern foods and additives should be on everyone's list of items to avoid:

Highly refined sugars

The tendency in Western health communities to vilify all sugars does not fit with TTM theory. Natural unprocessed sugars are considered extremely useful medicines for hydration, and honey is used in countless medicines for a variety of purposes. This said, sugar intake should not be excessive, and highly refined sugars should always be avoided. The worst culprits include white crystalized sugar and high-fructose corn syrup, which are poisons to the body, overtax the metabolic system, and can lead to diabetes and liver or kidney problems. Use honey, grade B maple syrup, raw sugar, stevia, jaggery, or palm sugar as a substitute.

Bleached white flour

This over-processed food is extremely common in modern Western cuisine. Bleached flour not only can contain high levels of toxins but it has been stripped of almost all of its nutritional value (which then is added back in to make "enriched flour). White flour breaks down rapidly into sugar in the digestive system, and leads to the same conditions as excess sugar consumption. Furthermore, white flour is exceedingly difficult for the digestive tract to handle, leading to sluggish digestion, and depletion of the Wind and Fire Elements. Use unbleached white or whole wheat flour instead.

Milk

Milk is another case of an over-processed food. Much of the nutritional value in raw milk is neutralized by the pasteurization and homogenization process, and then has to be added back in after processing. The vitamin D touted by the dairy industry is usually an additive, and can just as easily be ingested through other foods or supplements. The dairy industry is also a leading user of hormones and antibiotics, which many health advocates believe can enter the human system and cause long-term damage to the endocrine and immune systems. Raw or pasteurized cream-top milk from grass fed cows is largely considered a better nutritional choice, although there are some concerns with its safety and local laws vary. You can also use kefir or yogurt, goat milk, or dairy substitutes such as homemade almond or rice milk.

Hydrogenated Oil

With a chemical composition close to plastic, hydrogenated oils are some of the most dangerous and non-nutritive substances in our foods. Hydrogenation is usually done for consistency or texture, as food companies believe it makes the food appear less greasy than whole oil. The process renders beneficial oils useless by the body, and hydrogenated oils are immediately stored as fat.

Hydrogenated oils also lead to heart and circulatory disease. Look for hydrogenation-free products, as these are widely available.

Artificial Colors, Flavors, Preservatives, and Other Additives

The typical Western consumer eats piles of chemical food additives in every meal. These unnatural ingredients are both unhealthy and unnecessary. Read the nutritional labels on your food purchases, and look for alternative, 100 percent natural foods. Remember that in TTM, everything you put into your mouth has a transformative effect on your body and mind. It is therefore essential that you eat mindfully, trying to maximize the natural, healthy ingredients in your diet and minimize the artificial additives.

When examining the typical American diet, you may notice that many of us eat items from the above list in every meal. In fact, some "American classics"—such as a hamburger, fries, and Coke from a fast-food chain, or Froot Loops and milk for breakfast—are almost totally made up of these items. Individuals should try to limit the amount of junk food intake, especially the very young and the very old, who lack the strength to deal with these toxins. According to the Thai theories of the Elements and Tastes, overeating these foods can result in serious disorders. Most of the above items are Sweet foods, which deplete the Wind Element, leading to depletion of digestion, sexuality, and mobility, and increasing the effects of aging. Because of their refined processing, these foods affect the body much more strongly than natural foods, which is what you should use if you are looking for the Sweet flavor.

Another consideration that we might keep in mind, although Jīvaka did not mention it and it is more of a modern concern, is the long-term global effects of our dietary choices for the sustainability and health of our planetary environment. For example, while they are not the health hazards that some of the foods above are, items such as palm oil, musk, shark's fin, and so forth are directly related to environmental destruction and the endangerment of wild animals. We believe that foods that are environmentally unsustainable should be avoided as much as possible. This is not only a moral but also a health issue, as personal health becomes ever more difficult to maintain on a damaged planet.

There has been considerable controversy over the safety and ethics of genetically modified foods lately, which is an issue that deserves special mention. While GMOs are commonly sold in the United States, they are restricted in other countries with stronger food safety laws. Even if it is definitively proven that GMOs are safe to eat, there are considerable ethical problems that have yet to be worked out, including the environmental impact and social costs of corporate monopolies on seed supplies. For these reasons, we are currently of the belief that GMO foods should be avoided.

Dietary Regimen for Health and Longevity

While TTM provides guidelines for incorporating the Six Tastes into everyday dietary decisions, it is important to remember that some Element fluctuation is natural with seasonal shifts, time of day, and age. It is not recommended that anyone undertake extreme dietary change in reaction to these natural shifts. In general, it is also not suggested that you undertake a wholesale change all at once, as this will lead to further Elemental imbalances. Instead, you should lean slightly away from certain foods and slightly toward others on a seasonal basis, or to accommodate for an imbalance. For instance, it is normal and appropriate that most people become slightly more Fiery during the summertime, slightly Windier in the fall, and slightly more Watery in the winter. We are living organisms, not static objects, so movement in our Elemental balance is simply a side effect of being alive. The following guidelines are therefore suggestions for incorporating certain Tastes, not rigid rules.

Age

- Children up to age 16 should consume more Sweet, Bitter, and Sour foods to ward off childhood illnesses, colds, and coughs.
  Recommended herbal supplements for children's diet: anise, honey, gooseberry, lemon, licorice, lime, longan, milk, pineapple, tamarind.

- Young adults aged 16–32 should consume more Astringent, Salty, Bitter, and Sour foods for vitality, healthy blood, and bile.
  Recommended herbal supplements for young adult diet: aloe juice, bitter gourd, chrysanthemum, gooseberry, green tea, lemon, lime, orange rind, pineapple, pomegranate, seafood, tamarind.

- Adults aged 32 and older should consume more Spicy/Hot, Bitter, Salty, and Astringent foods.
  Recommended herbal supplements for middle-age adult diet: aloe juice, basil, bitter gourd, black pepper, cardamom, cayenne, chrysanthemum, cinnamon, clove, garlic, ginger, green tea, jasmine, lemongrass, lotus, orange rind, pomegranate, seafood, turmeric, all bitter greens.

- Adults aged 50 years and older are recommended to use special herbs as part of their diet for strength, longevity, and the heart.
  Recommended herbal supplements for older adult diet (in addition to suggestions for those aged 32 and up): asafoetida, honey, jackfruit, papaya, safflower, sesame.

Season

TTM includes a number of different ways of connecting the seasons of the year with the dietary changes and herbal remedies one should consume. The most common of these systems counts three seasons. The advice for the three seasons are as follows:

- In the hot season, individuals should consume more Bitter, Astringent, and Sweet foods, which are cooling to the system and relieve Fire Element diseases.

- In the rainy season, one should ingest more foods of the Salty, Spicy/Hot, and Sour Taste, which alleviate the effects of Wind.

- In the cold season, Spicy/Hot (including the gentler Aromatic Pungent herbs) foods are recommended to stimulate the Fire Element.

Since most of the West has four, rather than three, seasons, some reinterpretation will be necessary if we are going to apply these principles to our own yearly cycles. TTM does have a Four Season System based on the lunar calendar, and the adventurous herbalist can attempt to correlate these dates with the Western calendar. In our opinion, however, it is easier to start by modifying the Three Season System for use outside Thailand. The hot season and cold season clearly correspond to our summer and winter, and many areas of the United States and Europe have what could be considered a rainy season in the springtime. Of course, some flexibility and judgment will be required when using these recommendations outside of Southeast Asia.

In addition to these dietary recommendations, there are traditional herbal remedies associated with each season as well. These are described in detail in the list of medicinal recipes in Chapter 5.

Time of Day

A further breakdown of Taste recommendations can be given according to the time of day as follows:

MORNING: Eat more Sour foods, as they dissolve phlegm
MIDDAY: Eat more Bitter and Sour foods to calm Fire
EVENING: Eat more Spicy/Hot and mild foods to assist with digestion

Daily Dietary Supplements for Elemental Balance

There are certain Taste recommendations for daily intake depending on your core Elemental constitution (or which Element is agitated within you, if different). A little of the following should be consumed each day.

Excited Element	Eat a Little Every Day
Wind	Ghee, nuts, healthy oily things
Fire	Bitter things, such as bitter greens (kale, collards, dandelion, arugula, and so forth) and bitter melon. Also, cooling foods such as watermelon.
Water	Two glasses of hot water with lime, honey, and ground black pepper each morning before meals. Also eat sour, slightly diuretic foods such as roselle or hibiscus tea.
All Elements	Seven black peppercorns each morning, swallowed whole like pills. Some say this was the Buddha's medicinal recommendation for all people, and maintains general health regardless of your Elemental balance.

Thai Recipes for Health and Harmony

Rich in spices and covering a wide gamut of flavors, Thai cuisine is noted for its often surprising combination of tastes. A Thai curry will be Spicy/Hot, Sour, and Sweet. A dessert may be Sweet and Salty at the same time, with a Fragrant/Cool twist. This interesting and unusual combination of flavors makes Thai food one of the most sophisticated cuisines in the world.

There are several reasons why tropical cultures around the globe usually develop more flavor-laden cuisines than their temperate counterparts. One reason is simply that a wider variety of food is available year round. Another reason is food preservation. All pre-modern societies used such techniques as smoking, pickling, fermenting, and drying to preserve food, but in hot climates where food spoils quickly, these methods of preservation were elevated to a high art form. Throughout the equatorial regions of the world, where spices are more plentiful, one still finds the frequent use of such herbs as garlic, ginger, and chili to aid in food preservation. In Southeast Asia, a wide range of fermented and pickled foods is still consumed, especially in rural areas, where refrigeration is a more recent development. The Thai diet includes many such foods, including mangoes pickled and rubbed with chili, dried bananas preserved in honey, fermented fish paste, and other strong-tasting delicacies that are highly stimulating, bizarre, and sometimes even distasteful to the Western palate.

Another reason for the liberal use of spices may be their medicinal qualities. In the tropics, where the climate is more conducive to bacterial, fungal, and viral infections, it seems only natural that the cuisine would include larger quantities of antibacterial herbs and spices. Not only do many herbs prevent bacteria from spoiling the food, but they are a type of daily "food therapy" to ward off illness. To give an example, Thai tom yum soup is an excellent remedy for intestinal trouble and the common cold. The main ingredients in the soup (galangal, kaffir lime leaves, garlic, and chili) are herbs that are known for their decongestant and antibacterial properties.

The following are recipes for Thai dishes that particularly embody the principles of "food therapy." These dishes are common throughout Thailand, and unless otherwise noted these recipes come from our own kitchen experimentations.

In all of the recipes below, you can feel free to experiment and make substitutions for unavailable ingredients. For vegetarian/kosher, use tofu, tempeh, or seitan instead of meat, and vegetable stock. Instead of fish sauce and shrimp paste, use soy sauce, salt, or Bragg's Liquid Aminos. In recipes that call for palm sugar, use evaporated cane juice or raw sugar as a substitute if unavailable. Before you decide that an ingredient is unavailable, though, be sure to check and see if there are any Asian grocery stores in your neighborhood. The ingredients used in our recipes below should all be available with a little bit of detective work.

Appetizers

THAI LETTUCE WRAP (MÎANG KAM เมี่ยงคำ)

A favorite appetizer in Thailand, this is a cornucopia of medicinal herbs, a fun hors d'oeuvre, and an instant "taste of Thailand." It is a perfect example of a dish that truly uses all six Tastes and that can balance all the Elements in the body. Amounts for individual ingredients for this dish are not given, but a handful of each should suffice.

Use any or all of the following. (Asterisks denote core ingredients):
* Peanuts, roasted and salted
* Coconut, shredded and toasted
* Lime, chopped into ⅛-inch segments, including the rind
* Shallots, chopped small
* Fresh Thai chili peppers, minced (remove seeds for milder spice)
* Garlic, minced
- Ginger, shredded
- Raisins
- Starfruit, diced
- Cashews, roasted and salted
- Wild pepper leaf (use culantro, sesame leaf, chard, or spinach as substitute)

Dipping sauce ingredients:
- 1 part honey
- 1 part water
- Cilantro, diced
- Dried cracked red chili to taste

Typically, this dish is served by placing smaller bowls with each individual ingredient around a central plate of betel or lettuce leaves. Allow your guests to make their individual creations by wrapping the leaves around any or all of the other ingredients.

· · · · ·

YOUNG MANGO WITH SWEET CHILI SALT (MÁ-MÛANG PRÍK GLEUA มะม่วงพริกเกลือ)

This tasty snack is sold by street vendors all over Thailand. It is excellent for dissolving phlegm and has blood-purifying properties.

- 1 unripe mango, peeled and sliced into ¼-inch thick, long slices
- 2 tbs (30 ml) sea salt
- 2 tbs (30 ml) palm sugar
- 2 tsp (10 ml) dried chili flakes

Mix sea salt, sugar, and chili flakes. Dip your young mango slices and enjoy!

. . . . .

CHICKEN PANDANUS (GÀI HÒR BAI DTOIE ไก่ห่อใบเตย)

The pandanus palm is used in herbal medicine as a heart tonic, a fever-reducer, and a diuretic. In this dish, the leaves are not eaten, but their use in the cooking process infuses their medicinal qualities into the chicken. (This recipe is used with permission from the Chiang Mai Cookery School.)

- 7 oz (190 g) chicken breast, cut into twenty 2-inch pieces
- 20 pandanus leaves (nori seaweed may be used as substitute)
- 4 tbs (60 ml) roasted sesame seeds
- 1 tsp (15 ml) ground black pepper

Sauce Ingredients:
- 1 tbs (15 ml) light soy sauce
- 1 tbs (15 ml) tapioca flour
- 1 tbs (15 ml) sesame oil

Marinate chicken in sauce ingredients for half an hour. Add sesame and black pepper, and mix well. Wrap each piece of chicken in pandanus leaf, and secure by tying a knot with the leaf. Heat oil on medium heat in wok. Fry chicken or tempeh or tofu pieces for 5 min, until cooked. Drain on paper towels, and serve with chili sauce below.

. . . . .

SWEET THAI CHILI SAUCE (NÁM PRÍK WĂAN น้ำพริกหวาน)

A great accompaniment for some of the dishes above, or any time you long for a spicy tangy dipping sauce. Being sweet and spicy, this sauce good in moderation for Wind Element. (This recipe is from the Chiang Mai Cookery School.)

- 3.5 oz (100 g) cilantro root, chopped finely
- 9 oz (250 g) garlic, chopped
- 7 large red chilies, finely chopped
- 24 oz (700 g) palm sugar
- 5 oz (150 g) daikon or white radish, sliced in thin strips
- 1.5 cups (375 ml) vinegar
- ¼ (2 ml) tsp salt

Put all ingredients into a saucepan, and simmer on low heat for 20 min, until the sauce is thick, stirring occasionally. Once cooked, the sauce can be bottled and stored for up to one month in the refrigerator.

Main Dishes

"TOM YUM" SOUP (DTÔM YAM ต้มยำ)

One of the most popular dishes in Thailand, tom yum soup is the quintessential therapeutic dish, calling for a blend of spices that consists of many herbs recognized around the world as powerful tonics and antibiotics. This soup subdues the Water Element. It is a very soothing meal for intestinal trouble, and is especially beneficial for those suffering from congestion or cold without fever. Tom yum soup becomes tom kha with the simple addition of a ½ cup (120 ml) of coconut milk at the end. (This recipe is used with permission from the Chiang Mai Cookery School.)

- 10 oz (280 g) prawns, washed, peeled, and de-veined
- 3 cups (700 ml) chicken stock
- 6 cloves garlic, crushed
- 6 shallots, sliced
- 2 stalks lemongrass, white portion only, sliced into 1-inch pieces
- 10 thin slices of galangal, skin removed
- 7 oz (190 g) straw mushrooms, cut in half
- 8 cherry tomatoes, halved
- 20 small green Thai chilies, halved lengthwise (use less for milder spice)
- 3 tbs (45 ml) fish sauce or soy sauce
- 2 tbs (30 ml) lime juice
- 5 kaffir lime leaves, de-stemmed
- 2 tbs (30 ml) cilantro, chopped

Put stock, garlic, shallots, lemongrass, and galangal in a large stockpot and bring to a boil. Add mushrooms and tomatoes, and bring back to a boil. Add chilies, fish sauce, and kaffir lime leaves. Cook over medium heat for 2 min. Add prawns, and cook for 1 more minute. Remove from heat, and add lime juice. If adding coconut milk, add at the very end, after heat is turned off, to stop the lime juice from curdling it. Garnish with coriander before serving. (Serves 4.)

NOTE: *When serving this soup, one typically includes pieces of the lemongrass, galangal, and chilies that were used in cooking, but these should not be eaten.*

· · · · ·

THAI GREEN CURRY (GAENG KǏEOW WǍAN แกงเขียวหวาน)

A spicy, rich curry that is 100 percent Thai, and one of the country's most distinctive dishes. To simplify this recipe, buy green curry paste from any grocery that sells Thai food. Green curry is a good example of a Thai dish that incorporates all six medicinal Tastes. It is a well-balanced meal that is beneficial for all of the Elements, as long as it is not made overly spicy or sweet. (This recipe is from the Chiang Mai Cookery School.)

- 10 oz (280 g) chicken breast
- 3 tbs (45 ml) green curry paste (use only 2 tbs, if store-bought)
- 1 cup (240 ml) coconut cream
- 1 cup (240 ml) coconut milk
- 3 eggplants, cut into ½-inch pieces
- 2 tbs (30 ml) palm sugar
- 1.5 tbs (25 ml) fish sauce
- 2 kaffir lime leaves, de-stemmed
- 1 cup (240 ml) sweet basil
- 1 green chili, sliced
- 1 red chili, sliced

Green Curry Paste Ingredients:
- 1 tsp (5 ml) coriander seeds, roasted
- ½ tsp (2.5 ml) cumin seeds, roasted
- ½ tsp (2.5 ml) black peppercorns
- ½ tsp (2.5 ml) salt
- 1 tsp (5 ml) galangal, chopped and skin removed
- 3 tbs (45 ml) lemongrass, white part only, chopped
- 1 tsp (5 ml) kaffir lime leaf, chopped
- 2 tbs (30 ml) cilantro root
- 2 tbs (30 ml) shallots, chopped
- 1 tbs (15 ml) garlic
- 1 tsp (5 ml) shrimp paste
- 1 tsp (5 ml) turmeric, chopped and skin removed
- 20 small green chilies
- 1 cup (240 ml) sweet basil leaves

To make the curry paste, grind the dried ingredients into a powder with a mortar and pestle or coffee grinder. Mash all other ingredients with a mortar and pestle or in a food processor. Mixed the dry with wet ingredients, and set aside.

Put all but a couple of tablespoons of coconut cream into a wok, and simmer on medium heat for 3–5 min, stirring continuously. Add the green curry paste, and simmer for 1–2 min. Add chicken, and cook until white.

Add palm sugar, thin coconut milk, and eggplant, and bring to a boil. Cook 4–5 min, until eggplant is slightly soft. Add kaffir lime leaves and half of the basil leaves. Remove from heat. Garnish with chilies, remaining basil, and remaining coconut cream. (Serves 4.)

· · · · ·

THAI RED CURRY (GAENG PÈT แกงเผ็ด)

Green curry's sister dish, the equally famous Thai red curry. Again, to simplify preparation, you can buy red curry paste from any store that sells Asian foods. (This recipe is from the Chiang Mai Cookery School.)

- 9 oz (250 g) fish or butternut squash, cut into bite-sized pieces
- 3 tbs (45 ml) sesame or peanut oil
- 4 tbs (60 ml) red curry paste (use only 2 tbs, if store-bought)
- 3 cups (750 ml) coconut milk
- 2 large eggplants, cut into bite-sized pieces
- 4 oz (100 g) bamboo shoots, cut into bite-sized pieces
- 2 tbs (30 ml) fish or soy sauce
- 3 kaffir lime leaves, de-stemmed
- 2 large red chilies, seeds removed and sliced
- Basil leaves

Curry Paste Ingredients:
- 1 tsp (5 ml) galangal, skinned and grated
- 2 tsp (10 ml) lemongrass, white part only
- 1 tsp (5 ml) kaffir lime peel
- 1 tsp (5 ml) coriander root
- 1 tbs (15 ml) coriander seeds, roasted till brown
- 2 cardamom pods, roasted till brown
- 1 tsp (5 ml) salt
- 1 tsp (5 ml) black pepper
- 3 tbs (45 ml) chopped shallots
- 3 tbs (45 ml) chopped garlic
- 1 tsp (5 ml) shrimp paste
- 10 large dried red chilies, seeds removed and soaked in water for 10 min.
- 10 small red chilies

To make the curry paste, grind the dried ingredients into a powder with a mortar and pestle or coffee grinder. Mash all the other ingredients with a mortar and pestle or in a food processor. Mix the dry with wet ingredients, and set aside.

Fry the curry paste in oil in a wok over high heat for 3 min. Add coconut milk, and boil. Add eggplant and bamboo shoots, and simmer for 4 min. Add fish sauce, kaffir lime, and fish. Cook for 2 min, until fish is done. Serve garnished with large chilies and basil leaves. (Serves 4.)

• • • • •

BITTER GOURD STIR-FRY (MÁ-RÁ PÀT มะระผัด)

A tonic widely recommended by Thai herbalists, bitter gourd is beneficial for those with excited Fire Element, including fevers. The bitter gourd is accompanied in this dish by spicy herbs that encourage digestion and detoxification. However, if you are using this dish medicinally to treat Fire, you should omit or decrease the chilies. (This recipe is from the Chiang Mai Cookery School.)

- 7 oz (190 g) bitter gourd, chopped into ½-inch pieces (chopped zucchini, squash, or green beans may be substituted if you do not need the Bitter Taste)
- 3.5 oz (100 g) extra-firm tofu
- 4 tbs (60 ml) sesame oil
- 1 small onion, diced
- 6 cloves garlic, chopped
- 1 tbs (15 ml) shredded ginger
- 2 red chilies, sliced
- ½ cup (120 ml) chicken stock
- 2 oz (60 g) spring onions
- 2 tbs (30 ml) light soy sauce
- 2 tbs (30 ml) fish sauce
- 3 tbs (45 ml) oyster sauce
- 2 tbs (30 ml) sesame oil
- 4 tbs (60 ml) chopped basil

Prepare the tofu by boiling the slab in water for 10–15 min, until firm. Let cool, and crumble by hand. Heat oil in a wok or sauté pan over medium-high heat.

Fry garlic until brown. Add onion, and cook until soft. Add ginger, bitter gourd, tofu or scrambled eggs, sauces, chili, and 2 tbs water, and cook until bitter gourd is soft. Garnish with basil before serving. (Serves 4.)

• • • • •

PAPAYA SALAD (SÔM DTAM ส้มตำ)

Som tam, also known as "pok-pok" for the sound of the mortar and pestle when making it, is the most popular street-vendor meal in northern Thailand and is wonderful for stimulation of the digestion. The recipe calls for unripe papaya, which is a rich source of digestive enzymes, but this dish is delicious with unripe mango, raw zucchini, carrots, summer squash, or cucumber. When ordering this dish in Thailand, it may come garnished with fermented soft-shelled crab.

- 7 oz (190 g) unripe papaya, peeled and grated into thin strips (carrots and cabbage may be used as substitute)
- 3 cloves garlic

- 10 small green chilies
- ¼ cup (60 ml) green beans, cut into 1-inch pieces
- 2 tbs (30 ml) dried shrimp
- 2 tbs (30 ml) fish sauce or soy sauce
- 2 tbs (30 ml) lime juice
- 1 tsp (5 ml) palm sugar
- 4 cherry tomatoes, halved
- 2 tbs (30 ml) peanuts, roasted

Put the garlic, chilies, and beans into a mortar and pound with a pestle. Add papaya, and bruise. Add dried shrimp, fish sauce, lime juice, and palm sugar, and stir well. Mix in tomatoes and peanuts. Serve cold with sticky rice on bed of lettuce or cabbage. (Serves 2.)

· · · · ·

YOUNG JACKFRUIT CURRY (GAENG KÀ-NǓN แกงขนุน)

This spicy traditional northern dish is considered good for stimulating digestion and increasing appetite. Jackfruit is used to calm diarrhea, and many of the ingredients are considered beneficial for lower digestive tract issues, such as flatulence and indigestion. (This recipe is adapted from the book *Food for Health*, by the TTM Development Foundation.)

- 1 fresh young jack fruit, or two 10 oz cans young jackfruit (if using canned, be sure it is in water or brine, not syrup)
- 1 cup (240 ml) diced tomato
- 1 cup (240 ml) cha om (Thai acacia) leaves, finely chopped
- 9 betel leaves, chopped
- 7 oz (190 g) chopped pork ribs
- 4 c (950 ml) fresh water

Chili Paste Ingredients:
- 5 dried chilies soaked in water
- 1 tbs (15 ml) fermented fish
- 4 slices galangal
- 5 shallots
- 3 cloves of garlic
- 1 tbs (15 ml) salt

In a large mortar and pestle or food processor, grind all chili paste ingredients until a smooth paste is formed. Set aside.

If using fresh young jackfruit, smash lightly until soft. Peel and cut into small pieces, removing core and seeds. Soak jackfruit in lime juice to prevent discoloration. Set aside.

Boil water over high heat. Add pork ribs or bouillon. Add chili paste mixture and jackfruit, and simmer until well done, about 30 min. Stir in tomato. Add betel leaves and cha om just before finishing. Season to taste with salt or fish sauce.

· · · · ·

STIR-FRIED MORNING GLORY (PÀT PÀK BÛNG FAI DAENG ผัดผักบุ้งไฟแดง)

This delicious green dish is beneficial for not only the iron and calcium in the greens but also as a medicinal food that promotes good sleep and has a detoxifying effect on the body. Stir-fried morning glory is a popular dish throughout Southeast Asia.

This recipe is fairly standard throughout Thailand, with possible variances including using oyster sauce instead of mushroom sauce, chicken broth instead of water, and pounding the garlic and chilies together into a paste first for a stronger flavor. Note: The name "morning glory" is used for many plants. We are here referring to *Ipomoea aquatica,* which is available at many Asian groceries.

The Thai name of this dish translates as "red fire fried morning glory," named because of the flames that often leap up around the hot wok as the leaves are added.

- 6 oz (170 g) fresh morning glory, washed and cut into 2-inch pieces (use spinach as a substitute)
- 12–15 cloves garlic
- ½ (120 ml) cup raw cashew nuts
- 4 fresh small red Thai chilies
- 1 tbs (15 ml) palm sugar syrup (see instructions in compendium entry)
- 3 tbs (45 ml) soy sauce
- 3 tbs (45 ml) mushroom sauce
- 4 tbs (45 ml) vegetable oil
- ¾ cup (180 ml) water

This dish cooks very quickly, so be ready! Gently crush the whole garlic cloves so that they are still whole but slightly mashed. Put oil in a wok or pan over very high heat. When oil is very hot, but not yet smoking, add garlic and cashews and quickly fry until garlic is golden brown. When garlic turns brown, add all the other ingredients and flash-cook over high heat for about 30 seconds. Remove from heat, and serve with rice.

NOTE: *The speed of cooking is very important with this dish, as it can overcook quickly. Once the morning glory goes into the wok, it should not cook much more than 60 seconds at a maximum.*

· · · · ·

NORTHERN THAI GREEN CHILI DIP (NÁM PRÍK-NÙM น้ำพริกหนุ่ม)

Spicy dips (nam prik) are a traditional staple of northern Thai food. They are so common that one can find pre-roasted eggplant, garlic, shallots, and chilies sold skewered on sticks in the open markets, ready to be taken home and mashed together.

Often a meal will consist of one or two nam priks served with sticky rice, steamed vegetables, and pork skins. This recipe for green chili dip increases appetite and stimulates the body to sweat. (It is adapted from the book *Food for Health*, by the TTM Development Foundation.)

- 7 Thai long mild green chilies (you can substitute Anaheim chilies or any other long, light-green or yellow chili with some heat to it)
- 1 Japanese eggplant (optional)
- 5 cherry tomatoes
- 1 clove of garlic
- 5 shallots
- 2 tbs (30 ml) fish sauce
- 1 tsp (15 ml) salt
- 1 tbs (15 ml) scallion, cilantro leaves, and banana leaves coarsely chopped
- Lime juice to taste

Traditionally, the chilies, eggplant, garlic, and shallots are wrapped in a banana leaf and roasted. For modern preparation, first dry-roast the chilies by placing them in a very hot, dry cast iron pan.

Cook, pressing down on the chilies with a spatula, until blackened. Remove and set aside. Add the garlic, eggplant, and shallots to the pan, and repeat the process. Deseed the chilies, then mash all the ingredients together in a large mortar and pestle until you have a chunky thick paste. Serve with sticky rice, plenty of vegetables, and other items.

Desserts

THAI SHAVED ICE (NÁM KǍENG SǍI น้ำแข็งใส)

An easy dessert, and a soothing relief for sore throat, laryngitis, fever, and flu. A great substitute for ice-cream, and an instant refresher on a hot day. Not recommended for those with depleted systems or diseases of mucus. Also not recommended during cold weather or when women are menstruating, due to the depleting properties of chilled foods. At such times, a warming variation of this dish can be made by heating coconut milk, palm sugar, salt, and toppings, and eating hot.

Main Ingredients:
- Coconut cream (unsweetened)
- 1 tbs (15 ml) palm sugar, melted in 1 c (240 g) of water
- Shaved ice

Toppings (any or all of the following):
- Corn, cooked
- Barley, cooked
- Bananas, chopped
- Cantaloupe or honeydew melon, cubed
- Dates, de-pitted
- Raisins
- Taro, cooked and cubed
- Sweet potato, cooked and cubed
- Pumpkin, cooked and cubed

Prepare small bowls of shaved ice by adding 2 tbs coconut cream, 1 tbs of palm sugar water, and a pinch of salt. Top with any or all of the toppings.

· · · · ·

PUMPKIN IN SWEET COCONUT MILK (FÁK TONG GAENG-BÙAT ฟักทองแกงบวด)

There is a whole category of nourishing Thai desserts called *gaeng buat*. All of them involve cooking legumes or vegetables in sweet coconut milk. These desserts are nourishing for depleted bodies, young children, and the elderly. They are also healthy for those with agitated Wind or Fire Element, but should be eaten sparingly if you have agitated Water Element, including diseases of mucus.

- ½ (120 ml) cup coconut milk
- 1 cup (240 ml) water
- 2 cups (224 g) Thai pumpkin, skinned and cut into large bite-sized pieces
- ¼ cup (60 ml) palm sugar
- ½ tsp (2.5 ml) salt
- ¼ (cup 60 ml) coconut cream (optional)

Put coconut milk, water, salt, and sugar in a saucepan, and bring to a boil. Lower heat, and simmer while stirring, until sugar is dissolved.

Add pumpkin, and cook until done, being careful not to overcook the pumpkin, as it is not as nice if it is mushy. Turn off heat, and add coconut cream. Serve warm or cold. The milk will thicken a bit as it cools, so the dessert is thicker served cold.

Drinks

When making a tea drink, unless otherwise noted, it is best to use water that has had a moment to calm from boiling, or use water that was just brought to a simmer. Water at a high boil is too hot for some of the more fragile flowers in the recipes below.

· · · · ·

LEMONGRASS TEA (NÁM DTÀ-KRÁI น้ำตะไคร้)

This warming drink stimulates digestive Fire. It is beneficial for colds, indigestion, menstrual pain, and nausea.

- 10 stalks of lemongrass
- 6 cups (1 liter) water

Bruise the lemongrass by gently hitting the lower ⅔ of the stalk with a heavy object such as a pestle. Cut the lower ⅔ of the lemongrass stalks into 2-inch lengths, and place in a pot with the water. Bring to a boil, then reduce heat to simmer for 15–20 min, adding water as needed to compensate for evaporation.

Turn off heat, strain out lemongrass pieces. Sweeten as desired with a natural sweetener, such as palm sugar, evaporated cane juice, raw sugar, or honey. In Thailand, this drink is generally made very sweet. It can be drunk hot or cold.

· · · · ·

ASIATIC PENNYWORT TEA (NÁM BUA-BÒK น้ำบัวบก)

This green drink benefits conditions of the heart-mind—that is, the heart and the mind, which are considered a single function in TTM. It benefits both the physical heart and the emotional heart, as well as the brain and the mind. Asiatic pennywort can be found in many Asian food markets.

- 2 bunches Asiatic pennywort

Juice the Asiatic pennywort in a juicer and drink. Sweeten as desired with a natural sweetener, such as palm sugar, evaporated cane juice, raw sugar, or honey.

. . . . .

BUTTERFLY PEA FLOWER TEA (NÁM AN CHAN น้ำอัญชัน) *... with magic!*
Butterfly pea tea is sold by market vendors throughout Thailand. It is a beautiful blue- or purple-colored drink made from the dried butterfly pea flowers. It is said to treat depression, soothe the heart-mind, relieve stomach and menstrual cramps, and is known to be beneficial for healthy hair growth. In the West, you can grow your own butterfly pea vine, or you can order the dried flowers online.

- 1 handful dried butterfly pea flowers
- 2 cups (680 ml) simmering water
- 1 slice lime

Pour simmered water over the dried flowers and allow to sit for about 5 min. The water will turn a deep rich blue. Strain out the flowers, and squeeze the lime juice into the tea.

This is where the magic happens; your deep blue drink will turn vibrant purple. Add honey or palm sugar to taste (most Thais like it very sweet), and drink warm or chilled.

. . . . .

MULBERRY TEA (NÁM DTÔN MÒN น้ำต้นหม่อน) or
ROSELLE TEA (NÁM GRÀ JÍAP น้ำกระเจี๊ยบ)
Mulberry tea is beneficial to drink when you feel dehydrated or feverish. If you live where mulberries grow, you can harvest the leaves and berries and dry them to be used as needed throughout the year. Roselle tea or juice is beneficial for kidney stones and urinary tract infections. They are both delicious! If you cannot get roselle flowers, you may substitute dried hibiscus flowers as they are closely related.

- 1 handful fresh or dried mulberry leaves and berries or dried roselle flowers.
- 2 cups (680 ml) simmering water

Pour water over the leaves and berries, and steep for 10 min. Add a pinch of sea salt (especially if you are in a hot climate) and a natural sweetener. Drink hot or chilled.

. . . . .

SUGAR CANE JUICE (NÁM ÔI น้ำอ้อย)
While most people do not have the equipment needed to press the juice out of sugar cane, it is possible to purchase it in the West in many Asian and Latino grocery stores. Sugar cane is extremely beneficial for those suffering from dehydration resulting from heatstroke, fever, vomiting, and diarrhea. The Sweet Taste is medicinally rejuvenative, and fresh sugar cane juice will hydrate the body faster than simply drinking water.

· · · · ·

FRUIT SHAKE (PŎN-LÁ-MÁAI BPÀN ผลไม้ปั่น)

Fruit shakes can be tonics for health, strength, and vitality, with a stimulating effect on the digestion and a detoxifying effect on the body.

- 1 cup (240 ml) fresh pineapple
- 1 cup (240 ml) fresh longan
- 1 cup (240 ml) fresh papaya
- 1 tsp (5 ml) papaya seeds
- 1 fresh mandarin orange
- ¼ cup (60 ml) unsweetened coconut cream
- ¼ cup (60 ml) fresh sugar cane juice, honey, or palm sugar syrup (see instructions in compendium)

Squeeze juice from orange. Liquefy all other ingredients in blender. Drink cold.

· · · · ·

AVOCADO SHAKE (A-WOH-KAA-DÔH BPÀN อะโวคาโด้ปั่น)

A tasty and unusual drink found in Southeast Asia, an avocado shake will surprise you with its sweet, rich flavor, and it is packed with vitamins and beneficial fatty acids. At the street stalls, this is made with condensed milk. We prefer to use more healthful substitutes. If you omit dairy ingredients, it makes a great vegan milkshake.

- 1½ cup (360 ml) plain soy or almond milk
- ½ cup (120 ml) chipped or shaved ice
- 1 avocado
- 1½ tbs (22 ml) palm sugar, cane juice, honey, or raw sugar

Combine milk, ice, sugar, and avocado in blender. Serve immediately.

· · · · ·

BAEL TEA (NÁM MÁ DTOOM น้ำมะตูม)

Bael fruit is sliced and dried for making tea. It is balancing to the Elements, and soothes the stomach. It also is said to calm sexual energies. Bael tastes slightly like persimmon.

Simply pour boiled water over dried bael fruit and allow to steep for approximately 10 min. Drink hot or chilled, adding a natural sweetener, as you please.

Herbs in Cosmetics

While most of this chapter has concerned food, some mention should be made of the traditional place of herbs in cosmetics. Medicinal herbs are commonly used cosmetically for their natural toni-fying, rejuvenative, and skin-cleansing properties. Even today, in the largest cities in Thailand, some of the following traditional recipes enjoy more popularity than modern brand-name items. We recommend trying these natural recipes for a period of a few weeks, while abstaining from commercial products, in order to compare results. While a few of these recipes may take some getting used to, in a short time you will easily see the benefits of using home-made natural remedies instead of the massed-produced chemical alternatives. All of these preparations are 100 percent natural, and by using them you will lessen your exposure to the unnatural chemical compounds that are common in today's health and beauty preparations.

The following recipes are a mixture of traditional formulas and new discoveries inspired by Thai uses of herbs. In most of these recipes, we have purposely left out the proportions of the active ingredients in order to encourage experimentation. Have fun mixing your own products, and keep a log of what works (and what does not)!

. . . . .

BODY LOTION FOR DRY SKIN

Coconut, raw sesame, and olive oils are great moisturizers. (In fact, their main use in Thailand is cosmetic, and they are commonly sold in Thailand at the pharmacy as opposed to the grocery store!) Use olive oil for moderate to dry skin, coconut oil for severely dry skin, and sesame for severely dry skin that is also cold. Coconut oil has a cooling effect, and sesame oil has a warming effect, so you can also choose your oil based on the climate you are in.

Add 1 part fresh aloe gel to 2 parts oil, and apply thinly to the body. Allow 20–30 min for the nutrients to soak into the skin. Rinse off with warm water in the shower (don't use soap), and towel vigorously. For best results, an oil rub should follow a full-body dry-brush with natural fiber loofah or body brush.

. . . . .

BODY LOTION FOR OILY SKIN

Make the above recipe, substituting light olive oil. Add a splash of tamarind juice or kaffir lime juice and a dash of cider vinegar. Apply as above. The astringent action of the fruit juice in this recipe will cut through grease and cleanse the pores, while the cider vinegar helps maintain the skin's natural pH balance.

. . . . .

SHAMPOO SUBSTITUTE

An effective hair wash can be made by adding 2 handfuls of eucalyptus leaves (freshly mashed with mortar and pestle) to a quart of cold water along with one of the following ingredients:

- Jasmine
- Ylang ylang
- Rose
- Champaca

Let stand overnight, strain, and use as a rinse for hair. You will have to experiment with the quantity of eucalyptus. Use smaller amounts for dry hair, more for oily. Either mixture will keep up to 7 days, if refrigerated.

Eucalyptus is the cleansing agent in this shampoo, but Thai shampoos can also be made with kaffir lime, soap nut, neem, pomelo leaf, and other herbs. Try these if they are available in your area.

. . . . .

FACE AND BODY MIST

Cold-infused flower water is also perfect as a cleansing face and body mist. Soak any fragrant flowers (such as jasmine, rose, or ylang ylang) in cold water overnight, and strain. A standard spray-bottle is ideal to deliver an even mist to the face and body. When making mists, use distilled water for longer shelf life, and if using essential oils, be sure to use a moderate concentration to avoid irritation of face.

. . . . .

HOT OIL HAIR TREATMENT

Coconut oil, almond oil, or extra-virgin olive oil can give body and life to dry, brittle, or damaged hair. Mix in a splash of lime juice and mashed watermelon rind. Apply to the hair, making sure to rub the oil into the roots and scalp as well. Stand outside in direct sunlight for 10–15 min, allowing your hair to drink in the oil's nutrients and richness before rinsing off in the shower (but don't shampoo).

HERBAL FACIAL

To soften skin, eliminate acne, combat wrinkles, and ease topical irritations, the Thais use powdered ginger, a natural antibacterial and skin toner. Mix 2 tbs powdered ginger with 4 tbs of either:

- honey (for dry skin)
- kaffir lime juice (for oily skin)

Stir to a paste-like consistency. Apply to the face, taking care to avoid mouth and eye areas. For best results, let the mask sit 15 min. While rinsing with warm water, gently scrub for a mild exfoliant.

. . . . .

PAPAYA EXFOLIANT

Ripe papaya is a natural exfoliant and skin softener. Use fruit pulp, or apply the rind directly to the skin. Let stand for 15 min before rinsing.

· · · · ·

NONALCOHOLIC SKIN TONER

Lemon juice and tamarind juice can both be used as natural astringents, are safe to apply to the face, and confer the benefits of vitamins and minerals to the skin at the same time as they cut through grease and grime. A teaspoon of cider vinegar may also be added to help maintain the natural pH balance of the skin.

· · · · ·

TOOTH POWDER

While it may be initially strange for those of us who grew up on commercial toothpaste, natural tooth powder can be made that is just as effective, and it is 100 percent chemical free. Here are a few options:

Tooth Powder Recipe No. 1

- 3 parts neem powder
- 3 parts toothbrush tree powder (if available)
- 3 parts betel leaf powder
- 1 part clove powder
- 1 part salt
- 2 parts alum powder

Mix the powders together and store in air-tight container. Wet toothbrush, and dip in powder, then brush as normal.

Tooth Powder Recipe No. 2

- 8 parts neem powder
- 8 parts toothbrush tree powder (if available)
- 8 parts triphala powder
- 4 parts cinnamon powder
- 4 parts clove powder
- 2 parts star anise powder (optional)
- 1 part licorice powder
- ½ part salt
- ½ part alum powder

Mix the powders together and store in air-tight container. Wet toothbrush, and dip in powder, then brush as normal. This formula can be used as a mouthwash or gargle as well.

. . . . .

LIP BALM

Heat 1 part beeswax and 3 parts coconut oil over a low flame until melted. Remove from heat, and let cool in a metal or glass container. Use as necessary for dry, chapped lips, nose, and hands.

. . . . .

MOUTHWASH AND BREATH FRESHENER

Many of the herbs in this collection may be used as a light antiseptic mouthwash for combating oral bacteria, mouth sores, and bad breath. The following herbal teas can be used as a gargle after brushing teeth. Any combination of these may be used and may be mixed with other herbs or flowers (such as peppermint, jasmine, or lotus) for enhanced flavor:

- cinnamon
- ginger
- eucalyptus
- sea salt
- senna
- cloves
- paracress
- toothbrush tree
- galangal

. . . . .

NONTOXIC INSECT REPELLENT

A perfectly safe and non-irritating insect repellent that actually works!

- ½ tsp (3 ml) citronella oil
- ⅛ tsp (1 ml) jojoba oil
- ⅛ tsp (1 ml) tea tree oil
- ⅛ tsp (1 ml) neem oil
- ½ cup (150 ml) distilled water

Mix all ingredients in a spray bottle. Shake well before using.

. . . . .

SOOTHING EYE DROPS

A remarkably easy and useful recipe:

- 1–2 drops aloe gel
- 2 tsp (10 ml) saline solution

Mix well. Will keep in the refrigerator up to 7 days.

Herbs in the Household

Household products are among the most pervasive sources of harmful chemical toxins in our daily lives. The following are natural alternatives inspired by Thai herbal approaches, but not necessarily recorded in TTM texts.

. . . . .

COUNTERTOP CLEANSER

White distilled vinegar is a cheap and natural alternative for cleaning and disinfecting counter-tops, tables, and bathroom surfaces. Dilute 1 part vinegar to 2 parts water in a spray-bottle for easy application. Use a stronger concentration for problem areas, and add essential oils such as lavender or eucalyptus for added antibacterial action and a pleasant aroma. Pure vinegar may be used on carpets and upholstery to remove stains and odors, even from pets. Also try soaking fruits and vegetables in a light vinegar and water solution for 30 minutes to an hour before cooking to remove sediments, waxes, and pesticide residues.

. . . . .

COPPER TARNISH REMOVER

Lemon and lime juice are quite effective for removing tarnish and grime from copper, silver, and other metals. Cut fresh lemons or limes into wedges, dip into salt, and rub vigorously on tarnished surfaces. For particularly stubborn stains, scrub with a coconut husk or rough cloth. Rinse with water.

. . . . .

AROMATIC AIR FRESHENER

Put a drop or two of effervescent essential oil on a handkerchief, and drape over a lamp for 2–3 minutes. Small rooms will quickly be filled with a pleasant aroma without chemical perfumes or aerosol sprays, and you will benefit from the healing powers of aromatherapy at the same time. Perfect for freshening up the bathroom or creating a bit of ambiance in the bedroom. (For best results, try using thick musky or woody scents, such as patchouli or cedar.)

. . . . .

NATURAL MOTHBALLS

For an herbal alternative to the unpleasant odor of mothballs, make a sachet with dried cedar chips and lavender in a thin cotton cloth or cheesecloth. (A handkerchief with a few drops of essential oils may also be used.)

. . . . .

MOSQUITO-FREE ZONE

A popular method of keeping away mosquitoes in Thai villages is to keep a few handfuls of fresh citronella grass under the bed. The same principle can be applied in a modern setting. Use a few drops of essential oil of citronella in a diffuser or on a handkerchief, and you will sleep undisturbed.

· · · · ·

ALL-PURPOSE CLEANER

Baking soda is the perfect natural cleanser for almost any surface. Use it on stainless steel, silver, other metals, and porcelain. Works well in toilets, in ovens, and for unclogging drains. (Of course, it also cleans your teeth!)

· · · · ·

WINDOWS AND GLASS

While not an herb, we present the following window-cleaning option as an alternative to chemical cleaners, and as a point of interest. Newsprint is an effective cleansing agent; it can clean windows and other glass surfaces as well as any name-brand product, and without streaking. Spray water directly onto glass, and wipe dry with newspaper. It's that easy!

CHAPTER 4

Herbs in Traditional Thai Bodywork and Sauna

Sauna and Steam Bath

The sauna and steam bath play an important part in TTM. It is well known that these therapies promote general health, relaxation, cleansing of the skin, and detoxification by encouraging the release of toxins through the pores of the skin via sweating. In the Thai tradition, specific therapeutic herbs are added to the sauna or steam in order to enhance these effects, and in order to treat specific conditions such as respiratory diseases and infections, circulatory problems, skin disease, eye problems, sore muscles, colds, headaches, stress, anxiety, and other ailments. Steam baths are the preferred method, so long as the dampness is acceptable, as steam transports the aromas of the herbs well. Saunas, which are dry, are better for conditions with dampness, such as mucusy colds, which would not benefit from the added moisture of the steam. Traditionally, saunas and steam baths are used daily by Thai mothers in the weeks after giving birth, and there are herbs that are specifically used for this purpose. A regular herbal sauna or steam bath is also popular among the elderly, as it is considered good for promoting longevity.

Many traditional medicine providers in Thailand—TTM hospitals, clinics, and individual practitioners alike—have a sauna or steam bath, which is either used after massage or on its own. These saunas do not necessarily have to be of the cedar-paneled variety we know in the West. One massage teacher we knew in Chiang Mai built a small compartment in her backyard from sheet metal. This "hot box" had only enough room for a single occupant, who sat on a small wooden chair. Under the chair, a single electric steamer of the type used for cooking vegetables provided the steam. Even more simply, stove-top steam inhalation for colds and sinus infections can be employed by dropping herbs into a saucepan of boiling water. Leaning over the pot or steamer with a towel over your head is an ideal way to catch the aromatic vapors (although be careful to avoid being burnt by the hot steam or irritating your eyes).

Whatever type of inhalation therapy you are using, picking the right herbs can enhance your experience greatly. Herbs can come from any of the Four Taste classifications discussed below in this chapter. Add about 1 oz (30 grams) of most herbs to the steamer, but you may have to experiment with some herbs to get the perfect amount. (A few herbs are extremely potent, and should be used sparingly. For example, ½ tsp of camphor or less is all that is necessary for a strong effect.)

When using any type of sauna or steam bath, it is useful to remember that rhizomes, woods, barks, and seedpods often must be cooked for 10–15 minutes in order to release their therapeutic benefits, while more delicate flowers and leaves are damaged by heat in a fraction of that time. It is recommended to stagger the cooking so that all herbs reach their peak potency at the same time.

One word of caution: saunas or steam baths should not be used during pregnancy—or by those who are suffering from fever, hyper- or hypotension, or heart disease—without consulting a doctor. Also, saunas and steam baths are not recommended for anyone with agitated Fire Element or a generally Fiery constitution. Even if perfectly healthy, no one should use the sauna or steam bath for much longer than 10–15 minutes at a stretch. There is a very real possibility of overheating, and no matter how beneficial these herbs are, nausea, headache, irritated throat, and dizziness can occur from overexposure to vapors. It is recommended to take breaks and cold showers every 10–15 minutes, and to stop immediately if you experience any discomfort.

The following herbs are commonly added to the Thai sauna or steam:

Herbs		Therapeutic Action
Ginger Cassumunar ginger Zedoary	Turmeric Galangal Zerumbet ginger	General tonic for health and longevity, decongestant for colds and sinusitis, disinfectant for wounds or skin disease
Camphor crystals	Cardamom	Decongestant for colds, sinusitis, bronchitis or other lung infection, treatment for asthma and sore throat, stimulant
Tamarind leaf Soap nut	Kaffir lime leaf Neem	Cleansing of skin, opening of pores
Lemongrass		Increased energy, stimulation of mind and senses
Cinnamon bark	Ylang ylang flower	Stimulation of heart
Jasmine flower		Stimulation of heart, treatment for eye problems
Lotus flower		Tonic for heart, circulatory system, and blood

· · · · ·

SKIN CONDITIONER
Before entering the sauna, one of the following skin conditioners is frequently applied directly to the skin.

Astringents for oily skin:
- tamarind
- kaffir lime juice

Emollients for dry skin:
- honey
- powdered milk
- body lotions listed in Chapter 3

After finishing the sauna, rinse and towel dry, but do not use soap!

Herbal Inhalers

A common method of taking in the medicinal effects of herbs is through inhalation. This can be done traditionally in various ways, including steam and smoke; however, here we will describe a traditional Thai herbal inhaler (*yadom* ยาดม) that utilizes the crystals of camphor, menthol, and borneol. These traditional inhalers are found throughout Thailand, and can be bought at virtually any convenience store in the country. They are often sold in beautiful little silver canisters that can be carried easily in a pocket or purse, but they are just as effective in any nonporous vessel.

Herbal inhalers are beneficial for many conditions, including mental fog, respiratory congestion, nausea, faintness, headaches, anxiety, and even simply the need to get through a particularly odoriferous fish market.

· · · · ·

Three formulas are given here, all beginning with the following base:

HERBAL INHALER BASE FORMULA

- ⅛ cup (.75 g) dried whole green cardamom
- ⅛ cup (.75 g) dried whole mace (if you cannot find whole mace, use powdered)
- ⅛ cup (1 g) dried whole nutmeg
- ⅛ cup (.75 g) dried whole clove
- ⅛ cup (.75 g) dried whole black peppercorn
- ⅓ cup (2 g) menthol crystals
- ¼ cup (1 g) camphor crystals
- ¼ cup (1 g) borneol crystals (omit if not available)

In a small bowl, mix the three types of crystals. This step takes some time and is where the magic happens. If you mix them long enough, they will eventually become liquid. Once you have a liquid, set the bowl aside. In a mortar and pestle, crush the dried herbs (one at a time), until they are in tiny pieces, but not powdered. At this stage, add herbs from the specific formulas provided below. In a large bowl, mix well the dried herbs and the liquid from the crystals. Place the mixture in a lidded container.

Make sure that it is not packed tight; the container should be large enough that there is breathing room for the herbs. Store container in a dark, room-temperature space for 6 weeks. Do not open during this time.--

When ready, wrap approximately 1 tsp of the herbal mixture in small piece of cheesecloth, and place this inside of a small portable nonporous container (for example, a clean baby food jar, a glass vial, or a tincture bottle). Do not use plastic. Herbal inhalers are generally carried with you, to be used as needed.

· · · · ·

AROMATIC HERBAL INHALER FORMULA

This formula is beneficial for nausea, easing the mind, calming, and relieving dizziness.

- Add to the base formula above:
- ⅛ cup (.2 g) Szechuan pepper (also known as prickly ash)
- ⅛ cup (.75 g) cinnamon
- ⅛ cup (.75 g) star anise

· · · · ·

CITRUS HERBAL INHALER FORMULA

This formula is beneficial for lungs and sinuses, and general stimulation.

- Add to the base formula above:
- ⅛ cup (.2 g) dried kaffir lime leaf and/or peel
- ⅛ cup (.2 g) dried orange peel
- ⅛ cup (.2 g) dried lemongrass
- Any other aromatic citrus that you can find (such as pomelo, tangerine, grapefruit, etc.)

The total amount of dried citrus used should be equal to the total amount of the herbs in the base formula.

· · · · ·

MUSKY HERBAL INHALER FORMULA

This formula is beneficial for treating Wind imbalances, increasing appetite, and grounding, as the herbs in it are particularly earthy, both in smell and quality.

- ⅛ cup (.2 g) Szechuan pepper
- ⅛ cup (.75 g) cinnamon
- ⅛ cup (.75 g) star anise
- ⅛ cup (2 g) angelica

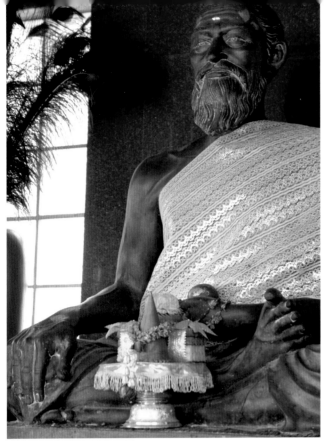

State of Jīvaka at Wat Phra Singh Temple in Chiang Mai.

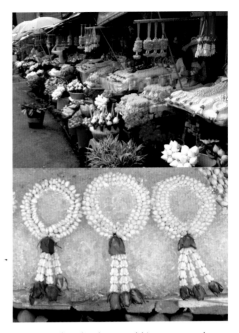

Devotional garlands are sold in many markets in Thailand. Many are later placed on statues of famous healers in order to show them respect and ask for their blessings.

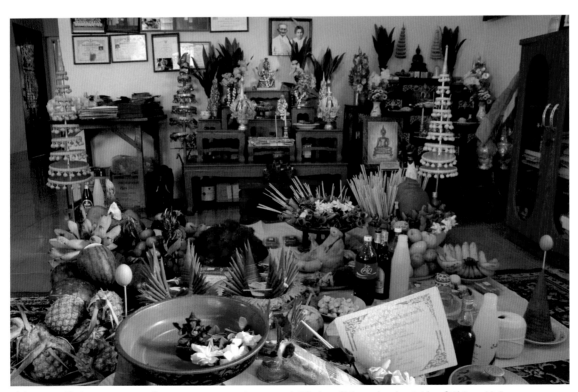

Elaborate offerings are set out for a ceremony at a Lanna-style Thai medicine school outside of Chiang Mai.

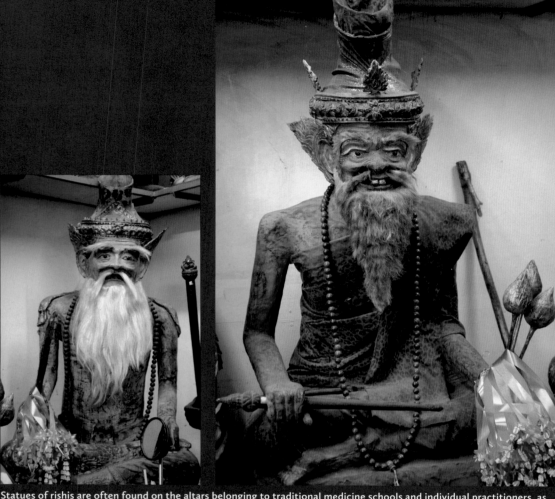

Statues of rishis are often found on the altars belonging to traditional medicine schools and individual practitioners, as they are revered for their role in the history of Thai medicine.

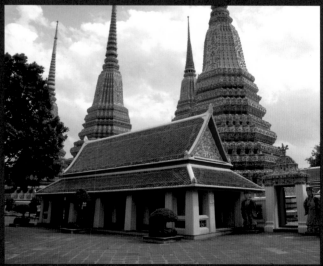

The medicine pagoda at Wat Pho in Bangkok houses a number of stone inscriptions depicting pressure points, sên, and herbal recipes.

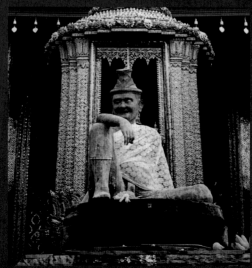

A statue of Jīvaka on the grounds of Wat Phra Kaew in Bangkok depicts him as a rishi.

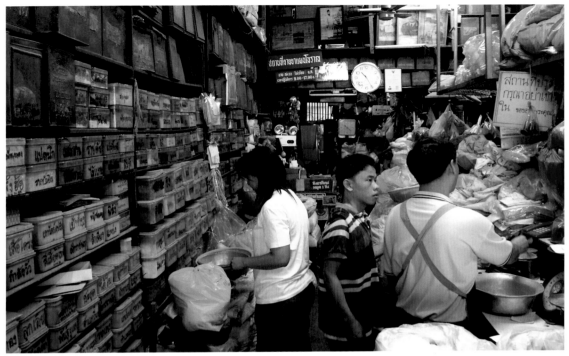
A bustling herbal wholesaler in downtown Chiang Mai.

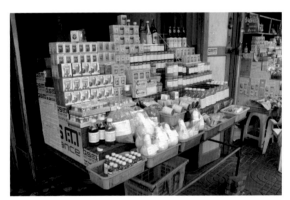
Street stalls selling herbal compresses and medicines outside of Wat Pho in Bangkok.

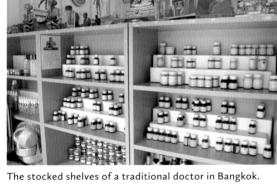
The stocked shelves of a traditional doctor in Bangkok.

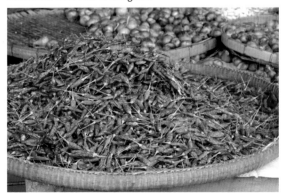
Chillis, garlic, and other common ingredients in Thai food are widely known for their medicinal properties.

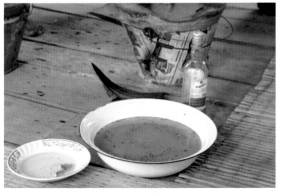
Medicinal oils used in the traditional practice of *yam khang* spirit-healing.

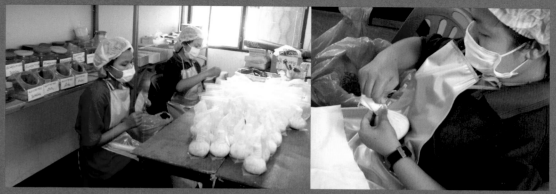

Making herbal compresses in Chiang Mai. (These women are wearing masks due to the potency of the camphor and other ingredients.)

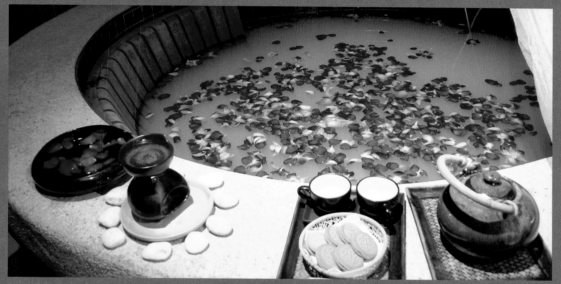

A combination of herbal baths, teas, and aromatherapy at a Bangkok spa.

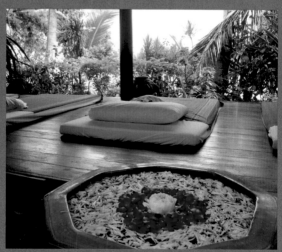

A platform is set up for Thai massage at a seaside resort in Koh Samui.

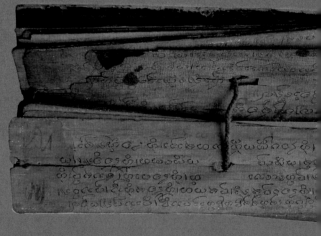

Texts about medicine were often transmitted by means of palm leaf manuscripts such as this one.

Body Layers and Four Taste System for the External Use of Herbs

When herbs are used externally, in balms, liniments, compresses, poultices, and plasters, the Four Taste system is employed. The Four Taste system uses Spicy/Hot, Astringent, Salty, and Sour. To better understand the use of herbs externally a bit of traditional Thai anatomy/physiology is needed.

In the TTM system, the physical body has five primary layers. From superficial to deep, these layers are:

1. **SKIN**, which can be broken down into the superficial skin, middle layer of skin, and deep skin.
2. **TISSUE**, which refers to the fascia, fat, and muscle tissue.
3. **SÊN**, or physical pathways in the body where movement occurs, such as tendons, ligaments, nerves, veins, and arteries.
4. **BONE**, including the joints.
5. **ORGANS**, which are further broken down as:
   Hollow organs, or those that connect to the external world (stomach, bladder, lungs)
   Solid organs, or those that do not connect directly to the external (liver, kidneys, spleen)

Understanding the layers is important when using herbs externally, because the herbs must penetrate to a specific layer in order to benefit a specific part of the body. Herbs used externally are not intended to reach the layer of the organs.

Four Taste System for External Use of Herbs			
Taste	**Permeates to:**	**Aids with:**	**Contraindications**
Spicy/ Hot	Permeates to layer of the skin	Relieves pain, removes stagnation, opens pores, enables other herbs to move to deeper layers	Inflammation, fever, rash, other symptoms of heat
Astrin-gent	Permeates to layer of skin and tissue	Binds wounds, relieves dampness, draws out toxins	Dryness, poor circulation
Sour	Permeates to layer of the tissue and sên	Moves blocked Wind, purges blockages in the sên	Excessive use can putrefy tissue
Salty	Permeates to the layer of the bone	Softens hardened tissue and masses that create stagnation, preserves tissue, heals adhesions	Open wounds

Knowing the layers of the body, the depth to which the Taste permeates, and what each Taste helps address is important when creating herbal formulas to be applied to the external body. For example, a typical Thai herbal compress (discussed below) will contain Spicy/Hot herbs such as cinnamon and clove to address the skin layer, Astringent herbs such as cassumunar ginger and turmeric to address the tissue layer, Sour herbs such as kaffir lime and lemongrass to address the *sên* layer, and salt to penetrate to the layer of the bone.

Herbal Compresses

Herbal compresses are frequently used in Thailand in conjunction with traditional massage or as a stand-alone therapy. While there are traditional formulas designed to be beneficial for a wide range of people that are commonly used in Thai bodywork, there are also practitioners who specialize in *luk pra kob* ลูกประคบ, diagnosing patients and formulating compresses for each individual. Cooling herbs may dominate a formula for an acute injury, overly excited Fire Element, or burns and rashes. Heating herbs increase energy flow, improve circulation, relax muscles, and stimulate nerves. Applied to joints and muscles, hot compresses can soothe soreness and increase flexibility. Applied to the abdominal region, they tonify and energize internal organs, and they are used in treatment of many internal disorders.

Hot herbal compresses are incredibly effective and have transformed many a Thai massage practice with their efficacy at releasing bound tissue and freeing movement (Wind Element) in the body. In addition, most people find the aroma to be appealing and relaxing. The herbs released in the air during the treatment serve to clear sinuses, and to simultaneously soothe and sharpen the mind. Hot herbal compresses are extremely nurturing and relax the recipient deeply, so they are an excellent choice for helping those who are stressed, anxious, or find it difficult to slow down. While Thai massage can be a complex modality that takes a serious commitment of time and dedication to master, using herbal compresses is a simple yet authentic Thai therapy that anyone can employ to bring healing to their friends and family. Plus, Thai herbal compresses integrate easily into a Western massage practice or many other modalities.

Making Compresses

To make a Thai herbal compress, chop or break fresh herbs into ¼–½-inch pieces, and mix in a large bowl. Alternatively, use precut and dried herbs. Lay out sections of cloth of about one square foot. (Any cloth may be used. Simple cotton muslin works well. We find that making herbal compresses is a wonderful way to recycle old yet clean sheets; simply cut them into one-foot squares.) Scoop a large fist-sized amount of the herbal mixture onto each. Wrap up the herbs, and secure the bundle with a rubber band.

STEAMED COMPRESSES
Your cooking techniques will differ for dried and fresh herbs, so it is important not to mix the two. If you use dried herbs, briefly dip your compress in water to wet the herbs before heating. Do not soak it; quickly putting it in and then pulling it out of the water will do.

Place bundles in an electric vegetable steamer or rice steamer. If you do not have a steamer, an acceptable substitute can be made by placing a metal colander inside a large saucepan or stock-pot.

Fill the pot with water up to, but not touching, the bottom of the colander, so that herb bundles will not become soaked.

If using fresh ingredients, steam the bundles for 5 min to begin to release the beneficial effects of the herbs. Since you will not be able to stagger the cooking time, you should begin to apply steam bundles as soon as they are hot, so as not to miss the benefits of the herbs that need less cooking time. Steam for at least 20 min if using dried herbs.

DRY COMPRESSES

While steam is generally the preferred method of heating compresses, dry compresses are optimal for damp conditions such as congestion in the lungs and sinuses, or water retention. To make dry hot compresses, the herbs can be heated on a dry skillet before being put into a cloth vessel (at home we use clean socks). Alternatively, a wrapped compress such as described above can be dampened to prevent fire, and then placed in an oven on low heat until reaching the desired temperature.

Compress Formulas

Choosing a harmonious combination of herbs for compresses will depend on a variety of factors, including the topical effects of the herbs, the mental effects of their aromas, and the preferences of the patient. Below are several of our favorite hot herbal compress recipes.

· · · · ·

TRADITIONAL WARMING COMPRESS

This is a standard formula that is beneficial for most people. It is extremely therapeutic for the tissue layer of the body, relaxing sore and stiff muscles and increasing circulation. Variations of this formula are found in most pre-made compresses that can be bought from Thailand.

- 3 parts turmeric
- 5 parts cassumunar ginger
- 2 parts galangal
- 2 parts lemongrass
- 1 part tamarind leaf
- 1–2 parts kaffir lime peel
- 1–2 parts kaffir lime leaf
- 1–2 tsp camphor
- 2 tsp rock salt
- 1 tsp borneol

· · · · ·

FRESH WARMING COMPRESS

This formula is a wonderful general compress that is beneficial for aches and pains, stagnation, and bound tissue. While a trip to an Asian market may be needed, these herbs should all be locatable in major Western cities.

- 2 parts galangal
- 1 part lemongrass
- 1 part mint
- 1 part shallots
- 1 part ginger
- 1 part turmeric
- 1 tsp camphor
- 1 tsp salt
- ½ part kaffir lime leaves or peel

· · · · ·

SALT DRYING COMPRESS

This easy-to-make compress aids with conditions of excess water, loose tissue, and loose joints. This is the only compress used on postpartum women, as it draws out toxins, dries the uterus, and assists the uterus back to its natural position. This compress is also beneficial for damp prolapsed tissue. Contraindicated during pregnancy.

This is a dried herb formula that is best made as a dry hot compress, although it can be steamed, if necessary.

- 5 parts rock salt
- 1 part cassumunar ginger (use galangal, if cassumunar is unavailable)
- 1 part long pepper
- 1 part cinnamon
- 1 part calamus
- 1 part turmeric
- ½ part myrrh

· · · · ·

COMPRESS FOR NERVE DAMAGE AND PARALYSIS

In Thailand, bodyworkers and herbalists often have great success with cases of paralysis, especially when working with stroke victims soon after the stroke event. Herbal compresses play a large role in the work that is done on these patients, combined with focused work on the *sên*. This compress can be used on any conditions of paralysis or nerve damage, including stroke, Bell's palsy, polio, and nerves damaged from long-term impingement.

- 5 parts rock salt
- 3 parts wax-leaved climber, broken up with mortar and pestle
- 1 part whole dried clove, broken up with mortar and pestle
- 1 part whole dried mace, broken up with mortar and pestle
- 1 part whole dried cardamom, broken up with mortar and pestle
- 1 part nutmeg, broken up with mortar and pestle

· · · · ·

SIMPLE DRY RICE COMPRESS

This is the modified solution we came up with in a pinch for family members suffering from congestion. Place the rice and salt in a dry frying pan and stir till hot, then bundle and use.

- 5 parts uncooked rice
- 1 part rock salt
- 1 part camphor, menthol, or eucalyptus

· · · · ·

COMPRESS FOR JOINTS

This compress contains the Thai herb gloriosa lily, a plant that has a particular affinity for the joints. The compress is beneficial for arthritis, gout, and various joint issues.

Equal parts:
- Black pepper
- Clove
- Frankincense
- Cinnamon
- Calamus
- Long pepper
- Gloriosa lily rhizomes
- White vinegar, enough to cover herbs

Grind the herbs gently with a mortar and pestle, until loosely broken. Place in a jar and cover with white vinegar such that the herbs are wet, but not drowning. Let sit for at least half an hour. Strain and place the herbs in compress cloth and steam as usual. Excess vinegar can be used as a liniment for the joints. You can make this formula and allow the herbs to sit in the vinegar for up to 3 months, taking them out as needed.

· · · · ·

ENERGY BOOST

For stimulation of mind, body, and energy. The hot herbs in this compress are penetrating and dissipating, so use them to soothe and relax tense, sore, pulled or over-worked muscles, open energy lines, and break up congestion. This was the basic formula used for massage patients by one of our Thai teachers.

- Ginger root
- Eucalyptus leaves
- Cinnamon leaves
- Kaffir lime rind and leaves

- Lemongrass
- Camphor crystals

· · · · ·

DRY SKIN HERBAL BATH

We like to use herb bundles in the bath tub, and any of the above recipes would work. However, the following combination of herbs has an especially relaxing effect, and is great for treatment of dry or chapped skin, sunburn, and dry hair or scalp. Add 2–4 unsteamed bundles to hot water, allowing them to soak for 10 min before getting in.

- Papaya leaves or rind
- Turmeric root
- Powdered milk
- Chamomile flowers

· · · · ·

HOT HERBAL PILLOW

Another trick with compresses is to use a hot bundle as a pillow. Lie on your back and place the compress right at the point where your neck vertebrae meet your skull. Another pillow may be placed under your lower back as well. As you lie on your back, allow your arms and legs to rest fully relaxed on the ground, and let your entire body sink into the floor. Breathe deeply and relax until the compresses have cooled.

Using Hot Compresses in Thai Massage

Thai bodywork is a complex healing modality that employs techniques ranging from muscle release point work to indigenous chiropractics (bone setting), and from intensive stretching to deep tissue compression. While Thai bodywork can address pain, injury, toxin release, and relaxation, the primary goal in Thai massage is to free movement in the body. Wind being the Element associated with movement, it is said that Thai massage frees the Wind. This is done by working on the physical pathways in the body where movement occurs, such as the tendons, ligaments, nerves, arteries, veins, and muscles. These are collectively known in Thai as *sên*.

The *sên* are frequently blocked by adhesions, or tight fascia and muscle tissue. While it is beyond the scope of this book to give instruction in Thai massage (for that purpose, see the companion book, *The Encyclopedia of Thai Massage*), one excellent tool for releasing these blockages is hot herbal compresses. For those who are unfamiliar with Thai massage techniques, hot herbal compress massage can be incorporated into an existing bodywork practice (including Swedish massage, hot stone therapy, or any other modality) or can stand alone as a whole-body therapy.

In Thailand, hot herbal compresses are used on areas of the body that are too tightly bound to be released easily through other massage methods, for deep relaxation, for pain relief where tightness is causing suffering, and in cases where sensitivity makes conventional massage techniques too painful (such as fibromyalgia, post surgery, elderly patients, and the very young). It is also the primary technique used in Thai prenatal and postnatal massage.

Steam or dry-heat the compresses as instructed in the previous section. When hot, wrap the bundle in a face towel so as not to burn yourself or your patient while using. Apply bundles directly to the skin or through the patient's clothes, taking care not to burn them (we typically test a steamed bundle on our own forearm before touching it to the patient's skin.) If applying directly to the skin, steamed bundles may be dipped lightly in room-temperature raw sesame oil or coconut oil before application in order to not burn. This also imparts the soothing and moisturizing benefits of the oil.

Exchange used bundles with hot ones from the steamer as necessary. Go through the bundles clockwise, so as to keep a regular rotation, and close the steamer lid in between to keep the bundles hot. (You may have to experiment a bit before being able to do all of this smoothly.) Bundles may be reused several times during the course of a massage, but you should use fresh ones for each patient. The cloth can be washed and reused.

When using hot herbal compresses, they must be used gently and quickly when they are very hot, but as they cool down enough to not burn they can be pressed into the body such that they provide compression as well as heat and herbal therapy. Compresses may also be left in one place as needed to let the heat really soak in. When stationary, the heat can become quite intense, so it may be necessary to place a small towel between the recipient and the compress so as to prevent burning. The following are some basic guidelines for using hot herbal compresses on a variety of conditions:

WEAKNESS

For weak and depleted recipients, begin at the extremities and work toward the core of the body. Try placing one warm compress on the stomach while you work, to warm the core.

RETAINING WATER

For recipients with excess water, such as edema, bloating, or postpartum, use the salt compress formula, and work from the extremities toward the core as you would with depleted recipients.

EXCESS HEAT

For recipients with excess heat, use herbs that have cooling properties, and do not use the compress when it is piping hot. Let it cool down a bit. Work from the core of the body out to the extremities.

LETHARGY AND FATIGUE

For recipients who are fatigued, lethargic, and weighted down, begin at the feet and work up toward the head using a faster, more energetic rhythm.

ANXIETY AND STRESS

For recipients who are anxious, stressed out, cannot stop thinking, or cannot relax, begin at the head and work your way down toward the feet using a calm steady rhythm.

PAIN

For recipients who have chronic pain and soreness, focus the compress specifically on the troublesome area. Hot compresses are generally not beneficial for acute, inflamed injuries.

LUNG CONGESTION

For recipients who are suffering from congestion in the lungs, use a hot dry compress and focus it over the chest and upper third of the back. Combine with gentle beating techniques over the upper third of the back to help break up stuck congestion.

Balms and Liniments

Balms and liniments are used extensively in Thailand. They are essentially the same thing; however, the herbs in a balm are held in a solid state with the addition of a natural wax, while a liniment is held in a liquid state either in alcohol or oil.

Many commercially available Thai balms and liniments claim multiple therapeutic benefits, ranging from relief of sore muscles to relief from congestion and insect bites. Most balms and liniments contain herbs for the first three or four layers of the body, and can be classified as either warming or cooling. Warming balms and liniments are beneficial for bound tissue, such as constricted or aching muscles. Cooling balms and liniments are beneficial for excess heat, and acute injuries that appear hot or swollen. While both can be useful for itchy insect bites, a cooling balm or liniment will bring more relief.

When using balms and liniments, it is important to vigorously rub them into the skin. Make sure that you don't just put them on superficially; take the time to massage them in. Then add more, and massage that in. The more balm or liniment you can get into the area, the better chance it has of delivering its beneficial properties.

· · · · ·

FRESH HERB WARMING BALM

This balm penetrates to the layer of the tissue, warming, healing, and soothing muscle and fascia. It is an excellent addition to any bodywork practice as it brings relief to aching muscles. Balms like this are used extensively throughout Thailand, and every herbalist has their own favorite version. Tiger Balm™ is a mass-produced and well-known example.

- 5 parts cassumunar ginger (substitute galangal, if unavailable)
- 3 parts galangal (if you used galangal above, substitute ginger here)
- 2 parts garlic
- 1 part chilies
- 2 parts lemongrass
- 3 parts turmeric
- 1 part basil
- 2 parts kaffir lime rind (optional)
- ⅓ part kaffir lime leaves
- 2 parts wild pepper
- ½ part camphor
- Raw sesame oil (you can mix or substitute with safflower if necessary)

- Beeswax, grated

Chop all herbs into small pieces. Deep fry each herb separately until crispy but not burned. If the oil burns, it must be discarded. Strain out and discard the herb, setting the oil aside. Fry the second herb as you did the first. After straining, combine its oil with the oil from the first herb. Continue in this manner until all herbs have been cooked and all of their oils have been combined.

Next, heat the combined oil and dissolve beeswax into it until enough has been added to obtain the consistency you desire. You can test the consistency as you go by putting a little of the warm balm on a spoon, and placing the spoon in a freezer for a few minutes to see how it solidifies. Once you have added all the beeswax you wish to add, stir in the camphor. Pour into desired container before the balm solidifies.

· · · · ·

FRESH COOLING TINCTURE

This fresh herbal tincture reduces inflammation, swelling, and stagnation. It is beneficial for acute injuries that have heat and inflammation.

- Equal parts plantain, mint, Asiatic pennywort, yanaang
- ½ cup menthol crystals
- Clear alcohol (80 proof minimum)
  Make sure that all herbs are fresh, clean, and have no water on them. Chop them up very small and place in a jar. Cover with alcohol and press the herbs down to release any caught air bubbles.

Cover with lid and let sit in a dark place for one month, shaking the jar daily to stimulate the release of herbal properties. After 1 month, strain the herbs and add the menthol crystals. Stir until dissolved.

Other External Herbal Formulas

HERBAL LICE REMOVAL

- ⅛ cup sugar apple seeds and/or 1 handful sugar apple leaves
- Coconut oil

Grind seeds and/or leaves and mix with coconut oil. Apply mixture to the hair and cover with a cloth or swim cap. Leave for 30 min. Comb out dead lice, and wash hair. Be very careful to avoid getting this mixture into your eyes.

. . . . .

CORIANDER EYE WASH

This infusion is beneficial for eye injuries, such as scratched cornea or sclera.

- ½ cup mashed coriander root (cleaned well to remove all sediment)
- 2 cups boiling water

Bring coriander root and water to a boil. Boil for 10 min, then simmer for 20 min. Remove from heat and cool before using as eye wash.

. . . . .

FOOT FUNGUS POULTICE

This formula is beneficial for various foot fungi including athlete's foot. It is also beneficial for warts.

- 3 parts fresh turmeric
- 2 parts fresh galangal
- 1 part fresh garlic

Mash all ingredients into a paste. If possible, soak foot in vinegar prior to applying poultice. Apply poultice to problem area. If needed, wrap in gauze to hold the poultice on. Leave for several hours or overnight. When combating a fungus, feet should receive as much direct sunlight as possible.

. . . . .

EAR OIL

This oil can be used for wax and fluid in the ears. Clove oil, in this instance, refers to oil that has been infused with clove, not essential oil. You can find clove oil at many Indian grocers, or make your own by breaking down dried cloves and allowing them to sit in raw sesame oil, in a warm dark place, for 3 months.

- 3–5 drops clove oil
- ½ oz raw sesame oil

Mix the clove and sesame oil, and put several drops inside your ear, lying on your side with the unaffected ear down.

CHAPTER 5

Internal Thai Herbal Medicine Therapies

Methods of Preparing Herbs

In this chapter, we discuss how to make infusions, decoctions, powders, and pills with herbs. The translation in Appendix 1 lists many methods for preparing and administering herbal medicines, including pickling, herbal soaks, oil preparations, suppositories, smoke inhalations and much more. We have chosen a handful of the most useful methods to share in more detail.

First, some preliminary notes and definitions:

- **MORTAR AND PESTLE**
  If you intend to explore Thai herbal preparations, you will want to invest in a good mortar and pestle. The small marble ones commonly available in Western herb shops are not adequate. These are mortar and pestles for apothecaries, and are designed for crushing small pills. They were never intended for kitchen use, and they simply will not suffice for Thai cooking or herbal preparation.

  Visit an Asian food market and look for a large stone mortar and pestle. (Clay ones are good for most food preparation, but are likely to break if used to break up tough nuts, barks, and heartwoods.) You will be delighted with your new crushing tool, both for cooking and herbal preparations.

- **SCALE**
  In all formulas given, parts are by weight, so you may also wish to invest in a digital kitchen scale.

- **ADJUVANTS**
  Sometimes, herbs are mixed with a second medicinal herb that complements the main ingredient. Adjuvant herbs may have beneficial secondary effects, may lessen certain side effects of the main ingredient, or may make the taste more palatable.

  For example, senna is a powerful laxative used for acute constipation, but it often causes intestinal cramping when used alone. In combination with ginger, though, senna has less pronounced side effects. In this case, ginger can be said to be an adjuvant, or "helping herb" for the main ingredient, senna.

- "VEHICLES"
  Vehicles are a type of adjuvant. These are herbs or bases that help direct the primary herb to the right place and assist it in doing its proper job. For example, lime moves the effect of the formula to areas of mucus, salt moves it to tissues and permeates the mucus membranes, flowers move it to the mind, honey moves it to the tissue and cuts through obstructions, and alcohol moves it to the *sên*.

- SWEETENERS
  Many of the herbal formulas discussed in this book call for a sweetener, which acts as an adjuvant or vehicle. However, the efficacy of most medicinal formulas will be altered with the addition of anything not in the original formula, including sweeteners; therefore, we recommend that you make the formulas as described here, without adding or subtracting any ingredients.

Infusions

An herbal tea or infusion is made by steeping plants in hot (never boiling) water for 2–3 min. Generally, infusions are made from delicate plant parts, such as flowers, leaves, shoots, or stems, which damage easily and therefore require a short exposure to heat for maximum benefit. They can also be made from many sturdier plants, such as ginger, licorice root, or cinnamon bark, which require a slightly longer steeping time. Some teas may be made by dissolving dried powders in hot water.

For herbal infusions, the dosage often varies depending on the age, strength, and severity of illness of the patient. Unless otherwise noted, the rule of thumb is to use one handful (about 1 oz or 30 grams) of fresh herb in one cup (8 oz or 250 ml) of boiled water. Halve that amount when using dried herbs. In any case, it is important to use enough of the herb to give the tea a strong flavor, but not so much that the consistency becomes thick.

· · · · ·

DIGESTIVE INFUSION

A gentle traditional remedy for indigestion and stomach cramps. Also great for clearing up colds, congestion, fever, and flu.

- 1 handful fresh basil leaves, flowers, and stalks
- 1 handful peppermint
- 1 tsp long pepper or black peppercorns

Steep ingredients in hot water for 3–5 min before drinking.

· · · · ·

TISSUE-SOFTENING INFUSION

This tea is good to drink 15 min before receiving massage as it will assist in softening the muscles and fascia. Massage therapists may wish to keep a batch made for clients. Note: All herbs in this recipe are dried, and parts are by weight.

- 2 parts Chinese hawthorn
- 1 part clove
- 1 part fennel
- 1 part lemongrass
- 1 part nutmeg
- 1 part haritaki
- 1 part cinnamon

Crush, but do not powder, the herbs with a mortar and pestle. Mix together. Place 1–2 tbs in a cup and cover with freshly boiled water. Steep at least 15 min before drinking.

· · · · ·

FRESH HERBAL INFUSION FOR MENSTRUAL CRAMPING

This can be drunk moderately throughout the day to alleviate pains associated with menstruation.

- 3 parts fresh lemongrass
- 2 parts fresh ginger
- 1 part fresh Asiatic pennywort
- Small pinch of salt

Place all ingredients in cup or teapot, and pour boiled (but no longer bubbling) water over them. Allow to steep for 10 min.

· · · · ·

ZINGIBER INFUSION

To stimulate digestion, cure flatulence, constipation, and indigestion; to decongest lungs, sinuses, and bronchi due to cold or allergies; to encourage regular menstruation; and for a general tonic and aphrodisiac.

- One 3-inch length of ginger root
- One 3-inch length galangal root
- 10 ml ginseng extract
- 1 tbs honey or bee pollen
- Juice of ¼ lemon

Boil ginger and galangal in 4 cups water for 10–15 min. Strain. Add ginseng, lemon, and honey before serving.

· · · · ·

ANTIOXIDANT INFUSION

For a vitamin C boost and detoxification. For smokers, drinkers, and those who live in polluted environments.

- 2 oz roselle or hibiscus flowers
- 20 clover blossoms
- 4 lemongrass stalks
- 1 tsp dried grated lemon or mandarin orange rind
- 3-inch cinnamon stick

Boil lemongrass, lemon rind, and cinnamon in 4 cups water for 10–15 min. Strain. Add hibiscus and clover, and steep for 2–3 min.

· · · · ·

INTESTINAL SOOTHING INFUSION

A soothing remedy for irritable bowel, stomach or intestinal cramps, indigestion, gastritis, and menstrual cramps. Gentle enough for children. Use honey or bee pollen as a sweetener.

- 2 tsp chamomile flowers
- 4 anise stars

Steep ingredients in hot water for 3–5 min before drinking.

Decoctions

Decoctions create a much stronger medicine than infusions. There are two ways to make medicinal decoctions. The first method presented here takes more effort, but produces a medicine that builds in strength over the course of several days of consumption. This not only results in a very powerful medicine but also allows your body a period of adjustment while receiving it. The second method is a simple and straightforward shortcut, if you are pressed for time or supplies.

Method 1:
Place the herbs in a large pot and cover with water 1 inch above the top of the herbs. Place lid halfway on the pot. Bring to a boil for 5–10 min, then reduce heat and simmer for another 15–30 min. Pour 1–3 cups of liquid through a strainer, to be drunk that day. Store the rest of the liquid and herbs in a jar in the refrigerator.

The next day, put the herbs and liquid back into the pot, adding water until it again reaches 1 inch above the herbs. Repeat the boiling and simmering process and again separate out the liquid that you will drink that day. Each day repeat the process, until the ninth day. After this do not boil anymore; simply drink the remaining liquid, one dose per day, until gone.

Method 2:
Place herbs in a large pot and add a large volume of water, perhaps 3 liters. Bring to a boil, then reduce heat and simmer until only about 1.5 liters remains. Strain and use.

In addition, any of the powder formulas discussed in the next section can be taken as decoctions. Buy whole dried herbs and loosely crush them to break them up instead of powdering them. Then, make a decoction according to the methods mentioned below.

. . . . .

TRADITIONAL DECOCTION FOR GENERAL HEALTH

This herbal decoction is beneficial for stagnant blood, bruising, and internal injuries. It is also good for strengthening the heart and the liver, prevents the accumulation of toxins that lead to disease, and improves the body's strength. Parts of plants are given in the traditional method.

- 1 handful Asiatic pennywort
- 1 thumb-length of galangal
- 7 slices of ginger
- Black pepper, as much as can be picked up between the thumb, index, and middle fingers
- 5 heads of lemongrass

Use the second decoction method, using 1 gal. (4 liters) of water to begin with, and simmering until there are 3 qts (3 liters) left. Strain out the herbs and store the liquid in the refrigerator. Drink 1 cup, three times a day. If using for internal injuries, add approximately 1 tbs of tasteless white alcohol (such as vodka) to each dose.

. . . . .

LIME COLD-CURING FORMULA

This tried-and-true formula is incredibly effective for stopping colds if taken at the onset, before the cold anchors in the body. Once a cold has set in, it must run its course. However, even in that case, this remedy will help the body to speed up the recovery process. Take at the first sign of sore throat or other cold symptoms. Credit for this formula goes to Ajahn Prasaht, a TTM practitioner in Northern Thailand.

- ½ lime, juiced (with or without pulp)
- 7 whole, dried black peppercorns
- 1 shallot, roughly chopped
- 1 clove garlic
- Pinch of sea salt

In a mortar and pestle, crush the peppercorns into powder. Add the shallot and garlic, and mash. Add lime and sea salt, and continue mashing. Eat the entire formula, but do not eat first thing in the morning on an empty stomach. If taking at onset of sickness, make the formula fresh and consume once or twice a day until certain that the illness is vanquished.

If already sick, make fresh and consume two or three times a day until well. Do not substitute onion for shallot, and do not add sweeteners. Because this formula tastes like a condiment, people are often tempted to combine it with rice or toast. This will make it less effective, as traditional medicine is based on the strength of the taste. For this reason it is important to ingest this formula (and all formulas) just as they are presented.

Powders

Many remedies that use dried seeds, nuts, or bark call for making a powder. This is traditionally done by grinding finely with a mortar and pestle. For the modern at heart, a coffee grinder works equally well, and you may want to reserve one for this particular purpose. Some powders (such as myrrh, for example) are almost impossible for the modern herbalist to make at home, but are readily available from herbal supply stores and Chinese pharmacies.

Making the powdered formulas below is very simple. Render each herb into a fine powder, then mix them all together. Following are some tips that will make the process go smoothly:

- Always use dried herbs.
- Whether using a mortar and pestle or an electric grinder, powder your herbs one at a time in small quantities. Remove powder before adding more of the herb to be crushed. Putting too much in at once seems like a time-saver, but ultimately makes the job of getting a fine powder more difficult.
- When using a mortar and pestle, don't be afraid to really have at it. New herbalists often have trouble simply because they are holding back their strength. Bash those herbs!
- If using an electric grinder, it is very important to stop and rest frequently in order to prevent the motor from heating up and thereby changing the properties of the herbs.

All of the formulas below are mentioned in the translation in Appendix 1, but we've given instructions on how to prepare them here.

· · · · ·

BENJAGOON เบญจกูล (*"Five Families" Element Balancing Formula*)
There are many variations of this remedy, which is said to correct the imbalance of the Elements and to cure any associated illnesses. (Benjagoon is a phonetic pronunciation that is helpful for pronunciation, but you may find this formula transcribed as "benchakun.") This formula should be taken during the transitional time between seasons, when people are most susceptible to Elemental imbalances and illness. Each herb in this formula is affiliated with a particular Element, and the measurements relate to the number of body parts associated with that Element. Herbs are listed in order from Earth to Space:

- 20 parts dried long pepper fruit (if unavailable, use dried nutgrass rhizome as a substitute)
- 12 parts dried wild pepper leaf
- 4 parts dried plumbago root (if unavailable, use dried black peppercorn as a substitute)
- 6 parts dried sakaan vine (if unavailable, use dried galangal as a substitute)
- 10 parts dried ginger

Powder and mix all ingredients. Mix 1 tsp of the powder with ½ cup of warm or hot water and a small spoonful of honey (when going into the cold season), jaggary (for rainy season), or rock sugar (for hot season). Take twice a day for 3–5 days. Do not take if overheated or feverish.

· · · · ·

TRIPHALA ตรีผลา (*"Three Fruits"*)

Triphala, trikatuk, and trisan are sister formulas that are well known in Ayurvedic medicine. They made their way to Thailand from India long enough ago to be mentioned in most traditional Thai medical texts, and are deeply integrated into Thai culture. Triphala is taken in the hot season, and regulates Fire Element.

- Equal parts bibhitaki, haritaki, amalaki

Powder and mix all ingredients. For general usage, take 1 tsp of powder with a little hot water.

· · · · ·

TRIKATUK ตรีกฏุก (*"Three Pungents"*)

Like triphala and trisan, this formula originates from India but has been used in Thai medicine for a very long time. It regulates Wind Element and is used primarily in the rainy season.

- Equal parts long pepper, ginger, black pepper

Powder and mix all ingredients. For general usage, take 1 tsp of powder with a little hot water.

· · · · ·

TRISAN ตรีสาร (*"Three Strong Medicines"*)

Trisan, like triphala and trikatuk, is the third of the sister formulas from India found in traditional Thai texts. The Indian formula typically uses cubeb (*Piper cubeba*) while the Thai substitutes sakaan, a different plant in the Piper genus. (In the West, either can be used, based on availability.) A "cold season medicine," this is a warming formula used to raise the body temperature and drive out winter chills. It regulates the Water Element.

- Equal parts plumbago, sakaan, wild pepper

Powder and mix all ingredients. For general usage, take 1 tsp of powder with a little hot water.

Pills

Pills are made by mixing powdered herbs together, and then combining with an adjuvant or vehicle. This can be as simple as water, or it might be honey, tea, lime juice, floral water, or rice water (to name a few). A pill is formed by either hand-rolling, or using a traditional tool. The pills are then dried and stored. Making herbal pills takes time and patience. Thai healers often spend this time chatting with friends or chanting healing mantras over the medicine they are making.

· · · · ·

TURMERIC HONEY PILLS
These pills are a gentle medicine that is good for inflammation, Wind in the abdomen, and liver support.

- 7 parts powdered turmeric
- ½ part powdered black pepper
- ⅛ part sea salt
- Local raw honey

Mix the powders, then add just enough honey to be able to roll the medicine into pills. Too much honey will make it difficult for the pills to hold their shape, and will extend the time needed to dry the pills. Lay out the pills on a screen, and place in the sun or in a very low-temperature dehydrator until dried. Keep in an airtight container. Take approximately 4 pills, two or three times a day.

Shelf Life of Herbs

The shelf life of a prepared herbal remedy varies depending on the substance and the method of preparation. The following guide is based on the climate of Thailand, which, due to the heat and humidity, causes some formulas to have short shelf lives. If you live in a cooler climate, your remedies will likely last longer than this.

Herbal tinctures in alcohol and essential oils	Up to 2 years
Dried barks	6–8 months
Dried seeds	6–8 months
Dried roots	6 months
Dry powders	3–6 months
Fresh herbs and liquid extracts	3–5 days (up to 7 days, if refrigerated)

With fresh herbs and liquid extracts, it is crucial to monitor shelf life carefully. Fresh plants lose their medicinal values rapidly, and it is important to keep in mind the length of time the herbs sat on the shelf before they were purchased. For example, "fresh" items bought at a typical supermarket may already be well past the 3–5 day period. Fresh herbs are always most effective when picked directly in a field or garden and used immediately, and most herbalists keep gardens at their homes for this purpose.

Our Thai Herbal First Aid Kit

In addition to common items such as bandages, isopropyl alcohol, iodine, and the like, our first aid kit at home includes many Thai remedies. Some of these are single herbs or compounds found in this book, while others are formulas that must be purchased. Homemade herbal preparations tend to be best, as the quality of mass-produced products is generally fairly low. However, if you are not able to acquire the herbs to make your own, or haven't yet found the time, having some ready-made formulas can be useful. With a little effort, you will find most of these online or at a local Asian market—although, whenever possible, we mention Chinese alternatives that are easier to locate in the West.

- **COOLING BALM OR LINIMENT** for inflammation, sprains, and other acute injuries. The formula is provided in this book, or you can easily find the Chinese equivalent, White Flower Liniment, at most Asian food markets and Chinese herb shops. Both cooling and heating balms and liniments will often state that they are useful for insect bites, inflammation, sprains, muscle pain, cramps and more. In general, cooling formulas will be better. Do not use these products on open wounds.

- **HEATING BALM OR LINIMENT** for sore muscles. A formula is provided in the previous chapter. There are many mass-produced heating balms available online if you search for "Thai balm." Many Asian food and herb shops in the West carry a gentle Thai warming balm called Monkey Holding Peach. If the balm states that it has ginger, cassumunar ginger, zingiber, pepper, or lemongrass, it is likely a heating balm. Do not use these products on open wounds.

- **PURPLE ALLAMANDA CAPSULES OR TEA BAGS** for poison. Poisoning can result from the overconsumption of alcohol, the consumption of any foods that one has an allergy or intolerance toward, or the consumption of harmful substances such as poisonous berries and mushrooms. While this is a rather benign herb, it should never be taken if you also take prescription medicines as it will clean them, along with the poison, out of your system.

- **ANDROGRAPHIS** capsules for oncoming sickness, such as a cold or sore throat. Andrographis is readily available in the West through health food stores, supplement shops, and online herb distributors.

- **HONEY** for sore throats and coughs caused by mucus. Best to use unfiltered raw honey if available.

- **GINGER** for upset stomachs. Young fresh ginger is best for children as it is mildest. Ginger can be made into tea for easy ingestion.

- **TURMERIC** for wounds and digestive issues. Turmeric can be found in bulk herb sections of Asian markets or in capsules.

- **HERBAL INHALER** for dizziness, faintness, brain fog, emotional upheaval, and clearing the sinuses. Use one of the formulas provided in this book, or purchase in a Thai market or online. Look for the ones that come in little silver- or brass-colored vessels.

- **LIME COLD-CURING FORMULA.** Keep limes, shallots, peppercorns, garlic, and salt on hand. The combination will stave off many a cold.

CHAPTER 6

A Compendium of
Traditional Thai Herbal Medicine

How to Use the Compendium

In this compendium, you will see an entry for each herbal medicine with the following information:

· · · · ·

ENGLISH COMMON NAME
[ALTERNATE COMMON NAMES]
Phonetic Thai transcription | Royal Thai transcription
ภาษาไทย

TASTE: *The medicinal Taste(s), mainly according to the Nine Tastes system (but sometimes with additional information drawn from other systems, from a range of teachers and texts)*
PART USED: List of parts used medicinally.

Internal Application
• How TTM texts and/or our teachers claim the herb should be used. This information is sometimes supplemented with additional points from our research in cultural or historical books, scientific papers, government websites, and comparative herbal traditions. Our sources are listed in Appendix 2. (This section is omitted when there are no known internal applications.)

External Application
• Based on the same sources as mentioned above. (This section is omitted when there are no known external applications.)

Notes on cultural practices, availability, and cautions, based on our own observations as well as the sources mentioned above.

Herb Names and Language

Each entry provides an English common name (sometimes several), as well as the Latin botanical name, the Thai name in Thai script, and the Thai name in two different transliteration systems.

While several different systems exist to transliterate the Thai language into the Roman alphabet, no one method has emerged as the clear favorite. As a consequence, newcomers to Thailand are often mystified by differences in spelling. The two systems that we find most useful are the royal transliteration system (as given in the software available from *http://pioneer.chula.ac.th/~awirote/ resources/thai-romanization.html*) and a phonetic transliteration system (as given by *http://www. Thai2English.com*). The royal system is useful when looking up Thai herbs in Thai herbal texts. However, the phonetic system will be more useful in attempting to pronounce the word (for instance when asking for an herb at a Thai herb shop).

When using the phonetic system, the tone marks described below are indispensable in helping you to pronounce the words properly. Thai is a tonal language, with five possible tones. Hence one word spoken with varying inflections can have up to five different meanings. For this reason, when using Thai words, you cannot ignore their tone.

The five tones are as follows:

1. **MID TONE:** Spoken in a normal voice, without inflection. These words have no tone mark in the transliteration.

2. **HIGH TONE:** Begin normally, but rise up at the end. Think of how you might say "Yes?" High-tone words are marked here with a ´ mark, above the word.

3. **LOW TONE:** Said deep in your throat and belly rather than in your mouth. This gives them a deeper, lower tone. Low-tone words are marked with ` .

4. **RISING TONE:** Begin with a fall, then rise up. Think of your word as traveling through the U of a roller coaster. Rising-tone words are marked with ˇ .

5. **FALLING TONE:** Sound a bit annoyed. Think about saying "come on!" for about the fifth time to someone who is making you late. Think of how the word "on" would sound, with a slightly long O sound, and bit of a whine that takes the word up, then down. Falling-tone words are marked with ^ .

Note for the Second Edition

The following compendium has been altered from the first printing of this book to reflect a more traditional understanding of Thai medicine. Hence it is now missing some herbs such as eucalyptus (introduced to Thailand in the 1950s), ginseng (imported relatively recently from China), and lemon (non-native and rarely found in Thailand). We have also removed a few herbs listed in the first edition for ethical reasons, such as musk, which comes from deer that are in some places endangered, and datura, which is a particularly dangerous plant if used unskillfully. We have also added several herbs not found in the original edition. With few exceptions, we have made sure that the herbs included in the second edition are: (1) mentioned in TTM texts we have read or been taught by our teachers, (2) able to be obtained readily outside of Thailand, and (3) found in a recipe, formula, or remedy mentioned elsewhere in this book. Or, they were simply so amazing that they had to be included.

The information we have read or been taught about the individual herbs that follow has been supplemented by our research in a variety of herbal reference books and other materials, all of which are listed in the bibliography at the end of the book. Please review the warnings in the beginning of the book before using any of the herbs in this compendium.

· · · · ·

ALOE
Aloe barbadensis/vera
wâan hăang jor-rá-kây | wan hang chorakhe
ว่านหางจระเข้

TASTE: *Cooling, Bitter*
PART USED: *Leaves, gel*

Internal Application: Traditional texts state that aloe is beneficial for treating ulcers in the stomach, and pulls out toxins from heat in the body. Aloe also strengthens the body. Among currently practicing traditional doctors, aloe is used for constipation and general weakness. Aloe has beneficial effects on the liver, spleen, uterus, and blood.

The gel of the aloe leaves is taken internally to regulate menstruation, for detoxification, for clearing up persistent lingering illness, for liver disease, and for chronic constipation. As it is a gently detoxifying laxative, aloe is a common adjuvant in the treatment of any infectious disease.

External Application: As is true the world over, aloe is used in Thai medicine to treat all kinds of topical burns. Traditional texts say that aloe nullifies the toxins or poisons from heat, and it assists in the healing of wounds. It is mixed with alcohol to treat abscesses, and it is protective to the skin. Aloe purges the tissues, is drying, and is also purifying. Yadam, the latex of the aloe plant, is used for constipation and bowel regularity.

The Thai name for aloe translates to "alligator tail plant." It is used by some Hill Tribes to combat epilepsy, seizures, and rabies. In internal Thai medicine, the form of aloe most frequently used is the dried powder. This can be obtained at some Chinese herb shops and well stocked herbal suppliers in the West.

· · · · ·

ALUM POWDER
Potassium aluminium sulfate
săan sôm | sansom
สารส้ม

TASTE: *Sour, Astringent*

Internal Application: Alum powder is a white crystalline salt. Traditional texts state that it is used to treat inflammation in the lungs and to move internal stones. In regards to reproductive health, alum is beneficial for treating abnormal discharge and gonorrhea, and for cleansing menstrual blood. Alum powder also serves internally as a diuretic.

External Application: Alum powder is beneficial in stopping bleeding. Alum powder is added to toothpaste or tooth powder to fight tooth decay, and to strengthen unhealthy or loose teeth. Alum treats wounds in the mouth, and it is also used to treat gum infections. It may be used on the skin for rashes, eczema, itching, scabies, ringworm, and other skin parasites.

Alum powder can be purchased at most Asian food markets in the West.

· · · · ·

AMALAKI
Phyllanthus emblica
má-kăam-bpôm | makham pom
มะขามป้อม

TASTE: *Sour, Astringent, Bitter*
PART USED: *Fruit*

Internal Application: The meat of the amalaki fruit is an astringent beneficial for dysentery and diarrhea. It treats jaundice and helps with digestion, as well as mucus and fever accompanied by Wind. Amalaki is soothing to the throat and treats cough. It is also used for cleansing the blood and treating hemorrhoids. One of the highest natural sources of vitamin C, amalaki treats scurvy. It is used in the traditional formula Triphala, which is found in traditional medicine across much of South and Southeast Asia. The fruit is a daily tonic for the brain, nervous system, blood, bones, liver, spleen, stomach, heart, eyes, hair, nails, teeth, and gums. Because of its detoxifying and antioxidant properties, amalaki is especially beneficial for those with frequent colds, low immunity, smokers, and those that live in polluted environments.

External Application: Amalaki is primarily used for internal medicine

In Thailand, the dried pickled fruits are sold in bags and eaten. Amalaki can be found in the West at some Asian food markets, including Indian food markets, and can also be found through Ayurvedic herb suppliers.

. . . . .

ANDROGRAPHIS [CHIRETTA]
Andrographis paniculata
fáa-tá-laai-john | fa thalai chon
ฟ้าทะลายโจร

TASTE: *Bitter*
PART USED: *Leaves*

Internal Application: Andrographis is beneficial in diseases of amplified Fire such as conditions with fever. It is used as a flu preventative, and it benefits patients with strep throat. Andrographis aids coughs, sore throats, and various upper respiratory conditions. It strengthens the immune system and fights allergies. As a bitter tonic, it is particularly stimulating for the liver, and increases production of bile. It has a beneficial effect on all liver and gall bladder disorders, as well as diabetes and hypoglycemia. Andrographis is a detoxifying herb, useful in cases of intestinal infection such as dysentery and other diarrhea, and in cleansing the blood. Andrographis is also used to relieve constipation, treat fever, and to reduce blood pressure.

External Application: Andrographis is primarily used as an internal medicine; however, it can be applied topically to especially strong skin problems, including infections.

The Thai name, fáa-tá-laai-john, translates as "the heavens strike the thieves." It is sometimes called the herb that kills 500 diseases, and it is used in Thailand extensively. When bird flu first hit Southeast Asia, Thailand nearly sold out of andrographis.

C A U T I O N: *While beneficial for many diseases, this is a very cooling herb and should be avoided with cold conditions.*

. . . . .

ANGELICA
Angelica sinensis
gòht chiang | kot chiang
โกฐเชียง

TASTE: *Chum, Aromatic Pungent, Mild, Fragrant/Cool*
PART USED: *Base of the stalk*

Internal Application: According to TTM texts, angelica treats fever. Beneficial for bronchial asthmatic cough and relieves hiccups, angelica also treats inflammation of the trachea, toxic mucus, and is a heart and blood tonic. Practitioners use angelica for building blood, cleaning the blood, and for treating bruises. It is beneficial for any type of premenstrual symptoms, including cramps, headaches, bloat, and muscle spasms. It is also effective in promoting regular menstruation when blocked. Angelica is used as a cold remedy, and against flu, fever, and generally low energy or low immunity. In small doses, it also stimulates the appetite.

External Application: Practitioners use angelica in herbal liniments for trauma, such as contusions, sprains, and strains.

Angelica is most easily found in the West at Chinese herb shops and online herbal suppliers. Chum is an untranslatable word indicating a strong "funky" taste that is often perceived as unpleasant. It is often musky, or pungent and odiferous.

· · · · ·

ANISE
Pimpinella anisum
tian sàt dtà-bùt | thian sattabut
เทียนสัตตบุษย์

TASTE: *Aromatic Pungent, Sweet, and slightly Heating*
PART USED: *Seed*

Internal Application: Anise is primarily used in conjunction with other herbs. Anise treats Wind having to do with the fetus (there are winds that turn the baby, and winds that move the baby out of the mother's body), and helps with shortness of breath and hiccups. If mixed with licorice it is good for treating cough.

· · · · ·

ASAFOETIDA [HING]
Ferula assafoetida
má-hǎa-hǐng | mahahing
มหาหิงคุ์

TASTE: *Chum, Heating*
PART USED: *The resin extracted from the root of fresh, living plants*

Internal Application: In TTM texts, asafoetida (also known in Thailand as "the devil's dung") expels Winds from the intestines, and thus treats abdominal problems, including bloating flatulence, tightness, gas pain, and stomachache. It is a tonic for the Elements, and it treats diseases of the nerves. Asafoetida also aids in digestion of food. A daily dose of asafoetida is reputed to be a tonic for the brain and the senses. It is also recommended for arthritis.

External Application: Topically, a poultice of asafoetida may be used to soothe arthritis and other joint pain.

Asafoetida and hing are commonly used names for this plant in the West. It can be found in Indian food markets, the bulk spice sections at many health food stores, and through online suppliers of herbs and Indian goods. Chum is an untranslatable word indicating a strong "funky" taste that is often perceived as unpleasant. It is often musky, or pungent and odiferous. Asafoetida is a spice with a particularly "chum" aroma.

· · · · ·

ASIATIC PENNYWORT [GOTU KOLA]
Centella asiatica
bua-bòk | buabok
บัวบก

TASTE: *Bitter*
PART USED: *Leaves, stem*

Internal Application: Asiatic pennywort is soothing to the heart and mind, relieving stress. It assists with mental clarity and calmness and brings emotional balance. Asiatic pennywort also reduces inflammation and heals contusions, and is beneficial for internal organs. It is used to treat psychological disorders, chemical imbalances of the brain, memory loss, Alzheimer's, and epilepsy. It is high in vitamin A, and is considered to be an excellent tonic for old age.

External Application: Asiatic pennywort reduces inflammation, soothes burns, clears bruises, and improves quality of skin. It also breaks up adhesions, heals scar tissue, and benefits acute tissue trauma. Asiatic pennywort treats skin conditions, such as staphylococcus infection and shingles, draws out poisons, and relieves bites. It is used extensively in cooling balms and liniments, and fresh herb poultices for acute injuries.

Asiatic pennywort is known to have a particular affinity for healing the heart-mind, and so is used for a range of ailments from heartache to cardiac troubles. Street vendors sell Asiatic pennywort juice out of clay pots. In the West, fresh Asiatic pennywort can be found at many Asian food markets.

· · · · ·

BAEL
Aegle marmelos
má-dtoom | matum
มะตูม

TASTE: *Astringent, Sweet, Heating*
PART USED: *Unripe fruit*

Internal Application: Bael treats the imbalanced Elements that are the cause of improper digestion. Bael is an appetizer, it increases strength, and it also expels gas. Bael is prescribed for any disorder of the intestines. The unripe fruit treats diarrhea, while the ripe fruit treats constipation, flatulence, and dysentery. The ripe bael fruit is traditionally used as a decongestant for the common cold, especially when there is excessive congestion of the lungs, as well as for tuberculosis and typhoid fever. Bael fruit is used for its stimulating properties in cases of exhaustion and convalescence from chronic disease or injury. Juice from the crushed leaves of the bael is given for respiratory infections, and decoction of the stem is said to be a useful antimalarial.

External Application: Bael leaves may be used topically as an antibacterial and antifungal for skin infections or wounds.

Bael is said to inhibit sexual energy and is for that reason drunk by monks at many monasteries.

• • • • •

BANANA
Musa spp.
glûay | kluay
กล้วย

TASTE: *Unripe banana is Astringent. Ripe banana is Sweet. The flower is Oily.*
PART USED: *Fruit, flower, peel*

Internal Application: According to traditional texts, the ripe fruit is an energy tonic. While it is not a laxative, it assists with the movement of the bowels. The unripe fruit is used for treating ulcers in the stomach as well as for diarrhea that contains undigested food. The banana flower reduces blood sugar levels, protects the intestines, and nourishes milk in lactating mothers. The ripe fruit of the banana is high in vitamins A and C, potassium, and carbohydrates, and therefore is useful for emaciation and wasting diseases. The ripe fruit is demulcent, the roots are diuretic, and the sap of the stem is Astringent.

External Application: While not the most effective option, in a pinch the peel of unripe bananas may be used for topical wounds to assist with healing.

There are 28 official species of banana in Thailand, with marked differences in size, shape, and flavor. Each has a different name in Thai, although glûay is useful as a general term. Some bananas are green when ripe, some are pink, others are mottled brown. According to traditional Thai cuisine, some are best in coconut milk, some are best raw, and some are only eaten soaked in honey and dried.

The flowers of the banana plant are similar in texture to cabbage and are added into salads or curries. The rest of the plant is utilized as well: the roots of the banana plant are converted into mulch, the fibers are woven into twine, and the leaves are used as plates and containers. A common method of cooking is to wrap ingredients such as rice, beans, fish, or vegetables in a banana leaf before grilling or steaming.

The banana is also a source of wine, vinegar, cloth dye, and flour. Pureed banana is a popular baby food, and batter-fried bananas are a favorite street-stall snack.

. . . . .

BASIL [THAI HOLY BASIL]
Ocimum tenuiflorum
gràprao | kraphrao
กระเพรา

TASTE: *Spicy/Hot, Sweet, Bitter*
PART USED: *Stem, leaves*

Internal Application: While basil has many possible medicinal uses, the one it is most often employed for is correcting digestive issues such as gas, indigestion, nausea, and vomiting. Holy basil is also a common ingredient in treatments for colds and flu. As an antispasmodic, it is useful for any stomach or intestinal cramping, including those caused by irritable bowel syndrome, peptic ulcer, and gastritis.

Holy basil is also used in treatments for easing headaches, cough, sinusitis, and arthritis. While the herb may be used to combat constipation, the seeds are more effective laxatives. Some Hill Tribes use basil in the steam bath or sauna for eye infections or pain, and topically as a poultice for fungal infections.

External Application: In topical formulas, basil reaches the level of the sên, specifically the blood vessels, where it increases circulation.

There are many other types of basil grown in Thailand including horapaa โหระพา *(usually simply called "Thai basil") and Thai lemon basil. Thai holy basil is most commonly used in medicine, hence this is the one we have focused on here. They are not always interchangeable.*

. . . . .

BETEL LEAF
Piper betel
phluu | phlu
พลู

TASTE: *Spicy/Hot, Toxic*
PART USED: *Leaves*

Internal Application: It is written in TTM texts that betel leaf treats tooth pain, sores in the mouth, and foul breath. It also alleviates gas, stomachaches, and diarrhea. Betel leaf also treats inflammation of the nasal passage and the throat.

External Application: Betel leaf is used externally for skin parasites, ringworm, and various fungi. It is also used for pain relief, and for treating bruises, itching, and rashes. It is beneficial for abscesses that come from tuberculosis. Applied topically to the chest, it acts as a decongestant and bronchodilator and is used in cases of congestion, difficult respiration, asthma, and diphtheria.

Betel nut is an addictive stimulant nut that is chewed throughout South Asia. It is generally mixed with a variety of other substances, including slaked lime, tobacco, and various spices, and has adverse health effects when used over time in this manner. The nontoxic leaf of the same plant can be found in the West in many Asian food markets.

• • • • •

BIBHITAKI
Terminalia belerica
sà-mŏr-pí-pâyk | samo phiphek
สมอพิเภก

TASTE: *Astringent, Sour, Sweet*
PART USED: *Fruit*

Internal Application: Bibhitaki treats mucus in the throat, and soothes the throat. It treats eye diseases and hemorrhoids, and is used as a laxative. Bibhitaki calms excitement of the Elements, treats fever (especially fever that affects the eyes), and is an Element tonic.

External Application: Topically, bibhitaki is antiseptic.

Bibhitaki is found in the traditional formula Triphala, which is common throughout much of South and Southeast Asia. It can be found in the West through Ayurvedic herbal suppliers.

• • • • •

BITTER GOURD [BITTER MELON]
Momordica charantia
má-rá kîî nók | mara khi nok
มะระขี้นก

TASTE: *Bitter*
PART USED: *Fruit, leaves*

Internal Application: The bitter gourd that is used in Thai cooking is usually má-rá, a larger variety. However for medicinal purposes, the smaller má-rá kîî nók (which translates as "bird-dropping bitter melon") is utilized. This melon is a bile tonic and blood cleanser. It increases appetite, strengthens the body, tonifies menstrual blood (treats scanty bleeding), treats the liver and spleen, and rids the body of parasites. Bitter melon is also beneficial for toxins arising from abscesses, and inflammation from various poisons, such as poisons from animals. It treats pain, Wind in the joints, and the juice helps conditions that affect the nerves of the mouth (such as Bell's Palsy).

This fruit is commonly used in rural Thailand to fight AIDS, hepatitis, and cancer, as well as other systemic diseases. It has particularly beneficial effects on diseases of the liver, spleen, and pancreas. The juice of the vegetable is a laxative and fever-reducer. Eaten daily as a bitter tonic, steamed bitter cucumbers are routinely suggested for the elderly, diabetics, hypoglycemics, and those with chronic disease or illness.

It has also been shown to increase insulin production, and to have anticarcinogenic properties. Bitter cucumber is recommended for sluggish digestion, dysentery, chronic constipation, and flatulence. It is also reputed to be beneficial for poor eyesight, and is high in the antioxidant vitamins A and C. Bitter cucumber is listed in the Wat Pho texts as an appetizer, purgative, anthelmintic, and as a cure for leprosy.

External Application: Topically, bitter gourd is antiseptic and treats infected and inflamed wounds. The juice of the bitter cucumber can be used topically on the skin and in the mouth as an antiseptic. The leaves are mentioned in the Wat Pho texts in topical remedies for tendonitis, swellings, infections, and headaches.

The form of bitter melon used in cooking is readily available at Asian food markets in the West; however, the smaller form used in medicine may be difficult to acquire.

·　·　·　·　·

BLACK PEPPER
Piper nigrum
prík tai dam | phrik thai dam
พริกไทย

TASTE: *Heating, Spicy/Hot*
PART USED: *Fruit (seed)*

Internal Application: Traditional texts say that black pepper treats Wind of the "central channel," and Wind that "feels like it is going to explode" in the abdomen—meaning that it treats gas in the abdomen. Texts also say that black pepper is an Element tonic, and that it treats sticky mucus and leukemia. Current practice uses black pepper for many cold conditions, and conditions in which Wind needs to be moved. It increases circulation, warms the body, and stimulates Fire Element.

External Application: Today, black pepper is used extensively by Thai herbalists in the making of balms and liniments. It is found in heating balms and liniments, as well as formulas for drawing liniments, joint pain liniments, and trauma liniments.

Swallowing 7 whole black peppercorns every morning is said to keep people of all Elemental makeups healthy. The Buddha is said to have prescribed this tonic to the forest monks who had little access to medical care. Black pepper, while not terribly hot to the tongue, is one of the hottest herbs once eaten internally. A bowl of black pepper soup will have you sweating profusely about 20 minutes after eating.

. . . . .

BORNEOL

Resin derived from a variety of trees, or synthetic compounding
pim-sǎyn | phimsen
พิมเสน

TASTE: *Bitter, Aromatic Pungent, Cooling*

Internal Application: Borneol is a heart tonic and stimulant.

External Application: Borneol is found in many Thai balms and liniments. It opens the pores and the mucus membrane, so it can assist in transporting other herbs through the skin layer of the body. Its vapors clear and relax the mind. The vapors also serve to clear the sinuses. Borneol can also be used to treat itching caused by insect bites, and thus serves in insect repellents.

Borneol can be found online and through some Asian herbal suppliers. In addition to the botanical sources listed above, borneol can be synthesized from a combination of camphor and turpentine. You can spot real borneol by its pink tint.

. . . . .

BUTTERFLY PEA

Clitoria ternatea
an-chan | anchan
อัญชัน

TASTE: *Cooling*
PART USED: *Flower*

Internal Application: Butterfly pea is taken internally to strengthen the hair, as well as to soothe stomach pains and cramps, and as a diuretic. Butterfly pea is also beneficial for depression and is soothing to the heart-mind. It is also beneficial for female reproductive health.

External Application: Butterfly pea is used externally for strengthening the hair, as well as for treating hair loss. The juice is used to treat eye diseases, and it is found in tooth powders for treating toothache.

Butterfly pea is used throughout Thailand to make a radiant purple drink that is commonly sold by street vendors. The botanical name for butterfly pea reflects the flower's resemblance to the female genitalia, and (because of the doctrine of signatures) this flower is said to benefit female reproductive health. Butterfly pea flowers are also used as food coloring and cloth dyes. Butterfly pea plants are available in the West, and you can purchase the seeds online. You can also purchase dried butterfly pea flowers online.

· · · · ·

CALAMUS [SWEET SEDGE, SWEET FLAG]
Acorus calamus
wâan nám | wan nam
ว่านน้ำ

TASTE: *Heating, Bitter*
PART USED: *Rhizome*

Internal Application: The primary use of calamus is to treat depression. It calms the mind, and acts as a nervine. Additionally, calamus is a stomachic traditionally used to treat indigestion, heartburn, gastritis, and hyperacidity, as well as to encourage appetite. Like most hot herbs, it is an effective cold cure and decongestant. It is used against cough, lung congestion, asthma, sinusitis, and fever. Calamus is considered to be a beneficial tonic and stimulant for the nervous system, especially the senses and the brain.

External Application: Calamus is found in liniments used to treat nerve pain and treats the sên.

Taken daily, calamus is said to enhance memory and sexual energy. In Western herbal medicine, smokers are told to chew the fresh rhizome in order to cause slight nausea, which aids in quitting smoking. Calamus is readily available at most Western herb shops.

· · · · ·

CAMPHOR
Cinnamomum camphora
gaa-rá-buun | karabun
การบูร

TASTE: *Heating, Toxic, Pra (an unpleasant taste)*
PART USED: *Crystals from the gum of the tree trunk*

Internal Application: Camphor is used internally only in small doses. It is a heart tonic, and it purges or expels Wind. It should be noted that while traditionally camphor was made from the sap of a tree closely related to cinnamon, today most camphor is synthetic.

External Application: Camphor is found in many topical herbal formulas, such as balms and liniments. Camphor opens the pores and mucus membrane, and thereby aids with absorption and moves Wind. Camphor also serves as a natural insect repellent, and its presence in balms and liniments frequently makes them beneficial for relieving itching associated with insect bites. The vapors of inhaled camphor open the sinuses and relieve congestion. Camphor, whether taken internally or inhaled, has both a stimulating and calming effect on the mind.

Because camphor burns without leaving any ash, it is commonly considered to be a metaphor for the enlightened mind, which vanishes into Nirvana without a trace. Camphor crystals are a common ingredient in most Thai saunas, from the traditional hospitals to the modern health clubs. Camphor can be purchased through various herbal suppliers in the West. You can tell real camphor from synthetic camphor by the color; real camphor has a slight off-white tint to it, while synthetic camphor is pure white.

C A U T I O N: Camphor is a mild adrenal stimulant and should only be ingested in a very small quantity.

· · · · ·

CANDELABRA BUSH [RINGWORM BUSH]
Cassia alata
chum-hèt-tâyt | chumhet thet
ชุมเห็ดเทศ

TASTE: *Bitter, Toxic*
PART USED: *Leaves, flowers*

Internal Application: The candelabra bush, like other cassias, is a laxative. It is primarily a purgative that treats parasites. It is mentioned in the Wat Pho texts as a cure for constipation, flatulence, diarrhea caused by intestinal parasites, and blood or mucus in the stools.

External Application: The leaves of the candelabra bush are used topically as an antiseptic and antiparasitic for treatment of ringworm, fungal and bacterial skin infections, and wounds.

Candelabra bush should not be used internally by children, or patients with inflammatory bowel diseases. It is said that candelabra bush can be "powdered together with zedoary and dusted on the body of a child who is difficult to rear, in order to prevent illness." It can be difficult to find in the West, but herbal suppliers can be checked.

· · · · ·

CARDAMOM
Amomum testaceum
grà-waan | krawan
กระวาน

TASTE: *Aromatic Pungent*
PART USED: *Seed*

Internal Application: Cardamom is known for its stimulating qualities and soothing effects on the gastrointestinal system. The tea is taken all over the world for cases of flatulence, bloated stomach, sluggish digestion, irritable bowel syndrome, and gastritis. In Thailand, varieties of cardamom are used to ease stomach pain and cramping associated with gastritis and indigestion. Cardamom is also widely used as a cough suppressant, as well as to treat colds, bronchitis, asthma, and laryngitis. Cardamom is an Aromatic Pungent, and is therefore calming to the Wind Element.

External Application: Cardamom is found in compresses and herbal inhalers.

· · · · ·

CASSUMUNAR GINGER [ASIAN GINGER, YELLOW GINGER]
Zingiber cassumunar
plai | phlai
ไพล

TASTE: *Heating, Astringent, Toxic*
PART USED: *Rhizome*

Internal Application: Cassumunar ginger expels menstrual blood, helps relieve numbness, eases stomachache, and treats Wind. It is beneficial for constipation, diarrhea, indigestion, and flatulence. Juice squeezed from the fresh rhizome is taken with salt for indigestion, dysentery, diarrhea, inflammation of the intestine, and injury to internal organs. It acts as a bronchodilator for treatment of asthma. Some Hill Tribes use cassumunar ginger to help new mothers recover after delivery.

External Application: Plai is used extensively in the external application of herbs in Thailand as it is especially beneficial for the skin and tissue layers of the body. Plai helps with inflammation and trauma. It is beneficial for coagulation, contusions, sprains, and strains.

Many plants in the ginger family are commonly called "Asian ginger", and turmeric is sometimes called "yellow ginger." Hence, it is important to make sure that you are getting the correct herb. Plai is very hard to find outside of Southeast Asia; however, it can sometimes be found frozen in Asian food markets in the West, and it is possible to grow it in warm climates.

· · · · ·

CASTOR OIL PLANT
Ricinus communis
lá-hùng | lahung
ละหุ่ง

TASTE: *Toxic, Heating*
PART USED: *Oil from the pressed seed and leaf*

Internal Application: Castor oil taken internally causes purging. It works to promote vomiting, and can be used as a laxative. The leaves are used to promote milk production. Expels Wind.

External Application: Castor oil is used in various liniments, as it has the ability to draw from the tissue layer of the body to the external skin. Purging.

C A U T I O N: The seed of the castor plant, if eaten, is deadly. Only the oil can be taken internally, and be sure that it is cold-expressed (hot-expressed castor oil is toxic).

· · · · ·

CAT'S WHISKER
Orthosiphon aristatus
yaâ nùat-maew | ya nuat maeo
หญ้าหนวดแมว

TASTE: *Tasteless*
PART USED: *Whole plant*

Internal Application: According to traditional texts, cat's whisker is used to eliminate urine, and it aids the excretion of uric acid. It also relieves problems with the kidneys and kidney or gall stones. Cat's whisker lowers blood sugar and blood pressure and treats infections in the urethra.

While it may be difficult to find cat's whisker being sold as a medicinal herb in the West, you can often find it being sold as an ornamental plant in nurseries.

C A U T I O N: Cat's whisker is contraindicated with patients with cardiac conditions.

· · · · ·

CHAMPACA
Michelia champaca
jam-bpaa | champa
จำปา

TASTE: *Bitter, Fragrant/Cool*
PART USED: *Whole plant*

Internal Application: The primary use of champaca is to treat the Subtle Winds and the mind. Tea from the champaca flower, like many aromatic herbs, is used to treat fever, chronic fatigue, and low immunity. It is also prescribed traditionally as a tonic for the heart, the nervous system, and the blood. Both the flower and the fruit are diuretic, antiemetic, fever-reducing (though only mildly), and are considered to be general tonics for the Elements. The leaf is used for neurological disorders, the bark of the stem reduces fevers, and the wood is a menstrual tonic.

External Application: Decoction of the champaca flower is applied to the temples to relieve headache. Decoction of the dried, ground root in milk is applied to abscesses.

· · · · ·

CHICKEN BONE [AROMATIC CHICKEN]
Chloranthus erectus
grà-dùuk gài [hŏm gài] | kraduk kai [hom kai]
กระดูกไก่ [หอมไก่]

TASTE: *Aromatic*
PART USED: *Stem, leaves, roots*

Internal Application: Chicken bone (called "aromatic chicken" in northern Thailand), is a plant used to treat fevers, sweating, headaches, and body aches. It is frequently mixed with cinnamon in formulas. It is also used to treat sexually transmitted diseases and muscle spasms.

External Application: Topically, chicken bone is used to treat inflammation and acute injuries.

This herb is not available in the West; however, it is a very useful herb for liniments that treat acute injury. If you happen to travel in Thailand, it can be found there.

· · · · ·

CHINCHONA
Cinchona calisaya
dtôn kwí-nin | ton khwinin
ต้นควินิน

TASTE: *Bitter*
PART USED: *Bark*

Internal Application: Until the advent of more potent synthetic medications, quinine derived from chinchona bark was the remedy of choice for malaria. It is still used for this purpose in isolated areas of rural Thailand, and throughout the world in places where modern antimalarial drugs are unavailable. In smaller doses, chinchona bark is also useful for cases of influenza, fever, and as a daily bitter tonic to promote health and longevity. Internally, chinchona is beneficial for leg cramps and restless leg syndrome at night, and is a mild muscle relaxer.

The Thai name for chinchona contains a phonetic transliteration of the word "quinine." This is not, in fact, a plant that is native to the area. It is nonetheless included here due to the significant role of antimalarials in the history of medicine in Southeast Asia.

C A U T I O N: In large doses, chinchona may cause headaches, dizziness, or stomach irritation. It may also cause uterine contractions, and should be avoided by pregnant women. It is toxic to some people.

· · · · ·

CHRYSANTHEMUM
Chrysanthemum morifolium
bayn-jà-mâat | benchamat
เบญจมาศ

TASTE: *Fragrant/Cool, Cooling*
PART USED: *Flowers*

Internal Application: Chrysanthemum relieves thirst and benefits the brain, liver, heart, and eyes. Therapeutically, chrysanthemum is used to treat all disorders of the liver and eyes, irregular or blocked menstruation, menstrual cramps, and PMS. It is also said to cure headaches and sore throat, to lower fever, and to calm the mind.

External Application: Topically, chrysanthemum treats inflammation and the eyes.

In Thailand, iced chrysanthemum tea is commonly sold by street vendors.

· · · · ·

CINNAMON
Cinnamomum spp.
op-choie | opchoei
อบเชย

TASTE: *Aromatic Pungent, Mild*
PART USED: *Bark, leaf*

Internal Application: Cinnamon moves and thins the blood. It regulates blood sugar levels and warms the body. Cinnamon also reduces fever and is said to treat paralysis. It is a stimulant for the kidneys, heart, and circulation, and is especially good in cases of chronic circulatory deficiency, hypotension, and chronic coldness. The tea also counters nausea and vomiting, soothes peptic ulcers and gastritis, and promotes regular menstruation.

External Application: In balms and liniments, cinnamon's ability to move and thin the blood aids the body's ability to rid itself of accumulated toxins. It is used in drawing formulas and other formulas that require increased mobility in the blood. The oil has a heating effect on the skin layer of the body, and is often added to balms and liniments in order to warm the skin so that herbs affecting deeper layers of the body can penetrate.

· · · · ·

CLOVE
Syzgium aromaticum
gaan phluu | kanphlu
กานพลู

TASTE: *Spicy/Hot, Aromatic Pungent*
PART USED: *Flower*

Internal Application: Clove treats abdominal problems, such as gas and pain, and clears the sên.

External Application: Clove is used externally in balms and liniments for pain relief, and to open the sên. It also purifies the blood. Clove is also used as an oral analgesic.

· · · · ·

COCONUT
Cocos nucifera
ma phráao | maphrao
มะพร้าว

TASTE: *Coconut water is Sweet and Salty; the oil is Oily and Sweet*
PART USED: *Nut*

Internal Application: Coconut water cleanses the body, treats dehydration particularly well, and is very cooling. The meat and milk of the coconut are nourishing, and coconut oil is used internally to draw toxins into the digestive tract, so that they can be expelled from the body.

External Application: Coconut oil is used extensively for external treatment. It is frequently the base for balms and liniments intended to provide cooling properties and to soothe external heat-related symptoms, such as dry rashes. Coconut meat is shredded and dried and then used in compresses for the face and for symptoms of heat.

The coconut palm is one of the most useful plants in Thailand. The fibrous husks of the coconut are used to make rope, mats, and brushes. Young green coconuts are prized for their sweet water, while the mature coconut is shredded, mixed with hot water, and strained to produce coconut cream.

C A U T I O N: Coconut water should not be consumed by menstruating women. It is too cooling for this time, and can even stop the menses.

• • • • •

CORIANDER [CILANTRO]
Coriandrum sativum
phàk-chee | phak chi
ผักชี

TASTE: *All parts used are Bitter, Sweet, and Astringent. The seed is also Aromatic Pungent. The root is also Fragrant/Cool.*
PART USED: *Seed, Root*

Internal Application: Coriander seeds are found in internal formulas designed to treat digestive issues, such as gas.

External Application: Coriander root decoction treats acute injuries to the eye.

Some people do not realize that coriander and cilantro (the Spanish word for coriander) are the same herb. In the United States, we use the word coriander to refer to the seed and the word cilantro to refer to the leaves; in most parts of the world, the word coriander covers the whole plant.

• • • • •

COSTUS ROOT
Saussurea lappa
gòht grà-dùuk | kot kraduk
โกฐกระดูก

TASTE: *Oily, Mild, Aromatic Pungent*
PART USED: *Root*

Internal Application: Costus root is a diuretic and an expectorant. It rids the body of mucus and water, and it has an affinity for the bones.

External Application: Costus root is used externally to rid the body of mucus and water. It also moves blood, and is found in drawing formulas (formulas applied externally for the purpose of drawing toxins to the surface of the body as a means of expelling them). Applied externally, it penetrates to the bone layer of the body.

The doctrine of signatures applies to costus root. Because it looks like bone, it is said to penetrate to the bone and to be beneficial for the bones. The Thai name grà-dùuk translates as "bone."

· · · · ·

CREPE MYRTLE [QUEEN'S FLOWER, PRIDE OF INDIA]
Lagerstroemia speciosa
in-tá-nin nám | inthaninnam
อินทนิลน้ำ

TASTE: *Bitter*
PART USED: *Leaf*

Internal Application: Crepe myrtle leaves serve as a diuretic and are beneficial for diabetes and diarrhea. It reduces blood sugar levels and is beneficial for painful urination, kidney and bladder stones, and treatment of venereal diseases.

Crepe myrtle grows wild in various Western climates.

· · · · ·

CULANTRO
Eryngium foetidum
chee fà-ràng | chi farang
ชีฝรั่ง

TASTE: *Bitter, Sweet, Astringent*
PART USED: *Root, seed*

Internal Application: Culantro is used as a laxative, and as a detoxifying purgative for malaria, allergic reactions, and poisonous insect bites. Another species, the amethyst holly (Eryngium amethystinum) is used for these purposes, as well as for increased immunity, chronic colds, and general longevity.

External Application: Culantro is used externally on allergic reactions and insect bites.

Culantro can be found in the West at Latino markets. The Thai name, phàk chee farang, translates as "foreigner's coriander." From this we can see that culantro is not native to Thailand.

· · · · ·

DAMASK ROSE
Rosa damascena
gù-làap-mon | kulap mon
กุหลาบมอญ

TASTE: *Fragrant/Cool*
PART USED: *Flower*

Internal Application: Rose is calming to the heart-mind as well as to the Subtle Winds. Rosewater is a common ingredient in South Asian desserts. Hot or cold, it may be used as a stimulant to counter low immunity, low energy, and chronic fatigue. The tea is a cholagogue, meaning that it aids in digestion by stimulating bile; assists in assimilation of nutrients; and encourages regular menstruation. Rose flowers are added to the traditional sauna or steam bath for eye disorders and infections, and for a relaxing effect on nervous disorders, anxiety, insomnia, tension headaches, and stress. Rosewater is often used as a medicinal binding agent for powdered herbal formulas that need to be rolled into pill form.

External Application: Rosewater and rose infused oils are calming to the heart-mind and soothe the Subtle Winds.

· · · · ·

DURIAN
Durio zibethinus
tú rian | thurian
ทุเรียน

TASTE: *The leaves are Chum. The fruit is Sweet and Heating. The roots are Bitter, Spicy/Hot, and Astringent.*
PART USED: *Leaves, fruit, roots*

Internal Application: The leaves of the durian tree treat jaundice, fever, and parasites. They also dry pus. The fruit heats the body, treats skin diseases, and dries up abscesses. It also expels parasites. The root treats fever and diarrhea.

External Application: Topically, durian treats wounds.

Durian is one of Thailand's most famous fruits. It is known as the King of Fruits and is often paired with mangosteen, known as the Queen of Fruits. Durian grows to enormous size and has a strong odor that deters many foreigners from trying it. (Chum is an untranslatable word indicating a strong "funky" taste that is often perceived as unpleasant. It is often musky, or pungent and odiferous.) Throughout Thailand, signs can be seen in taxis, buses, and other forms of public transportation that state "no durian," due to the smell. Durian contains high levels of tryptophan and is said to be slightly addictive, as it produces feelings of mild euphoria. It is also high in natural phytoestrogen, and for this reason is said to aid fertility. Durian is extremely high in many vitamins and minerals, in fact. Durian fruit can be found fresh or frozen in Asian food markets in the West. Always buy fresh for medicinal purposes.

CAUTION: Durian is one of the most Heating fruits available, and therefore must not be consumed with alcohol. In Thailand, they say that too much durian and alcohol together can be so overheating to the body it can be fatal. Studies have revealed that the sulphur content of durian interferes with the body's ability to process alcohol, and that while not necessarily fatal, the combination does at the very least leave people feeling unwell. Some doctors advise against eating durian during pregnancy as so much is still not known about this powerful fruit.

· · · · ·

EBONY TREE
Diospyros mollis
má-gleua | makluea
มะเกลือ

TASTE: *Heating, Astringent*
PART USED: *Fruit, root, bark*

Internal Application: The juice of the ebony tree fruit is used to purge tapeworms and other parasites from the intestines. The Wat Pho texts mention ebony tree root as a remedy for vomiting and nausea, and the bark as a remedy for emaciation or wasting associated with chronic illness.

Various Diospyros trees play the role of being the official provincial tree in different provinces of Thailand. Diospyros decandra is the provincial tree of Chanthaburi and Nakhon Pathom Provinces, and Diospyros malabarica is the provincial tree of Ang Thong Province.

CAUTION: It is widely held that combining ebony tree fruit juice with coconut milk may have toxic, even potentially fatal, results.

· · · · ·

FENNEL
Foeniculum vulgare
tian-kâao-bplèuak | thian khao plueak
เทียนข้าวเปลือก

TASTE: *Sweet, Aromatic Pungent*
PART USED: *Seed*

Internal Application: Fennel seeds are generally used in conjunction with other herbs in formulas that treat gas and Wind. Fennel is especially beneficial for treating Wind located in the center of the body, between the navel and the genitals.

. . . . .

FINGER ROOT [LESSER GALANGAL]
Boesenbergia rotunda
grà chaai | krachai
กระชาย

TASTE: *Spicy/Hot, Bitter*
PART USED: *Rhizome, leaves*

Internal Application: Finger root is used traditionally to treat stomach discomfort and peptic ulcers. It is beneficial for flatulence, indigestion, and sluggish digestion, and is used as a general diuretic. It is also used for tooth and gum disease, diarrhea, dysentery, and as a general diuretic. Tea made from the finger root leaves is employed in cases of food poisoning and allergic reactions to food.

Finger root is used in Thai cooking to flavor soups and curries, and can be found in some meat and fish dishes, where it serves to override the meat/fish odors. Finger root is available in the West at Asian food markets. If you cannot find it fresh, you can generally find it frozen. It is named for its fingerlike appearance.

. . . . .

FOETID CASSIA
Cassia tora
chum hèt tai | chumhet thai
ชุมเห็ดไทย

TASTE: *Bitter, Toxic*
PART USED: *Whole plant*

Internal Application: Decoction of foetid cassia seeds is preferred in cases of acute constipation and intestinal worms for its purging action on the bowels. It is also used to calm fevers, to lessen inflammation of the eyes, to lower high blood pressure and cholesterol, as a diuretic, and as a sedative. Decoction of the stem and/or root is also diuretic, and may be used topically to stop itching. Treats insomnia. NOTE: Seeds must be roasted until yellow smoke comes out before they can be used medicinally

External Application: Topically, foetid cassia is beneficial for itching and ringworm when mixed with oil. It also treats tick bites.

Foetid cassia grows wild on most continents.

. . . . .

GALANGAL [GALANGA]
Alpinia galanga
kàa | kha
ข่า

TASTE: *Spicy/Hot, Bitter*
PART USED: *Rhizome*

Internal Application: Galangal is used internally to stimulate digestive Fire, and is recommended for indigestion, flatulence, and stomach troubles such as diarrhea and nausea.

External Application: Galangal is used externally to nourish the tissue, improve circulation, and fortify the blood. It is often found in hot herbal compress formulas, balms, and liniments, and can be used in external healing poultices. Combined with other herbs it can be used as a fresh herb compress for fungal conditions, such as athlete's foot. Galangal can also be used for treatment of skin parasites and insect bites.

Galangal is the herb associated with the Wind Element and is found in the Element-balancing formula Benjagoon. While related to ginger, galangal is more aromatic and flowery. It is a key ingredient in many well-known Thai dishes, including tom yum, tom kha, and curries, and is one of the more common ingredients in Thai cooking. Galangal can be obtained from Asian food markets in the West. Look for rhizomes that appear lighter in color and have a plumpness to them despite their hardness.

C A U T I O N: *As stated above, galangal is used for external skin treatment in poultices; however, caution must be exercised as external use of fresh galangal can cause minor superficial burning.*

. . . . .

GARCINIA
Garcinia cambogia
sôm kàek | som khaek
ส้มแขก

TASTE: *Sour*
PART USED: *Fruit*

Internal Application: Used to heat the body. Dissolves phlegm, and reduces cough. Garcinia aids in weight loss by accelerating the metabolism of fats and carbohydrates. It has been the subject of numerous studies in the United States and Europe for use as a natural alternative to chemical weight-loss drugs. It has been found safe for long-term use, although some studies show it to have only a limited effect. It is now also being researched for antitumor and anticancerous properties. Garcinia is used in Thailand as a dietary supplement for suppressing the appetite. It is also used traditionally for constipation, edema, intestinal parasites, sluggish digestion, and for increasing body heat.

The Thai name translates as "Indian Orange," which gives us a clue as to its origin.

· · · · ·

GARDEN BALSAM [IMPATIENS]
Impatiens balsamina
tian bâan | thianban
เทียนบ้าน

TASTE: *Chum*
PART USED: *Leaves*

External Application: Externally, garden balsam treats eczema, skin ulcers, insect bites, allergic reactions, hives, sores, wounds, and bacterial infection of the skin and nails. The juice is applied to treat split nails. Garden balsam treats swelling, pain in the joints, and snake bites. Some Hill Tribes use the garden balsam topically for inflammation and low immunity, and an aid in the delivery of babies.

While finding garden balsam leaves suitable for medicinal purposes may be tricky in the West, you may be able to find it being sold as an ornamental. Chum (which is not listed in the main Taste systems) is an untranslatable word indicating a strong "funky" taste that is often perceived as unpleasant. It is often musky, or pungent and odiferous.

· · · · ·

GARLIC
Allium sativum
grà tiam | krathiam
กระเทียม

TASTE: *Spicy/Hot*
PART USED: *Cloves*

Internal Application: Garlic increases digestive Fire, and aids with digestive issues such as flatulence and indigestion. It cuts through mucus, and for this reason is beneficial for certain coughs and asthmas. Garlic builds immunity, fights infection, and is used as a purgative for internal parasites. It is a potent detoxifying agent, and is therefore beneficial in fighting liver disease, toxic colon, and in general detoxification of the blood and organs. In large doses, garlic has a purgative effect on intestinal worms and other parasites, and is used to prevent malaria and dengue. Other diseases that benefit from the use of garlic include arthritis, heart disease, gall bladder disease, fever, and cystitis. Garlic reputedly lowers blood cholesterol, lowers high blood pressure, raises low blood pressure, and is recognized in many cultures the world over as a stimulating aphrodisiac.

External Application: Used in balms, liniments, and poultices, garlic penetrates to the level of skin, moves Wind, and purifies the blood. Garlic is also beneficial in treating skin fungus and ear infections.

. . . . .

GINGER
Zingiber officinale
kǐng | khing
ขิง

TASTE: *Sweet, Spicy/Hot*
PART USED: *Rhizome*

Internal Application: Ginger is the quintessential panacea in the Thai herbal pharmacopeia. Ginger is a powerful stimulant, especially of the digestive tract. It is the herb of choice for stimulation of digestion, and is used to combat flatulence, indigestion, gastritis, peptic ulcer, diarrhea, sluggish digestion, nausea, and vomiting. Ginger tea is also used for colds, congestion, sore throat, fevers, nausea, seasickness, mouth sores, insomnia, heart disease, arthritis, irregular or blocked menstruation, chronic back pain, hemorrhoids, and beri-beri (vitamin B1 deficiency), earning it the reputation as a cure-all. Hill Tribe healers give ginger tea to mothers immediately following birth to promote health and rapid recovery. Ginger also acts as a galactagogue, meaning that it encourages production of breast milk. Ginger is used as an adjuvant in many herbal preparations in order to lessen side effects and increase the potency of other herbs, and is the most frequently used herb in this collection.

External Application: In balms, liniments, hot compresses, poultices, and plasters, ginger increases circulation, creates movement, and adds heat.

Ginger is associated with the Space Element, and is found in the Element-balancing formula Benjagoon. Dried ginger is the hottest form of ginger, mature fresh ginger is next, and young ginger is the least (the latter is therefore best for children).

. . . . .

GLORIOSA LILY
Gloriosa superba
dong deung | dongdueng
ดองดึง

TASTE: *Heating, Toxic*
PART USED: *Rhizome*

Internal Application: Gloriosa lily treats arthritis, joints, and gout. It is also used to treat sexually transmitted diseases and some cancers.

External Application: Used in liniments, compresses, and creams to treat joint pain, including arthritis. Extremely beneficial for the joints.

While gloriosa lily is not sold as a medicinal herb in the West, it can be purchased as an ornamental, and the rhizomes can be utilized. The doctrine of signatures applies here: the rhizomes have a bend in them that looks like a joint, and thus the plant is thought to be beneficial for joint care.

· · · · ·

GOLDEN SHOWER [PURGING CASSIA]
Cassia fistula
khuun | khun
คูน

TASTE: *The meat is Sweet. The flower is Bitter and Sour.*
PART USED: *Seed pod, flowers*

Internal Application: The sickly sweet, black, and sticky pulp surrounding the seeds of the golden shower is used traditionally as a laxative and expectorant. In larger doses, it is a purgative. Tea from the flower is also a laxative and a reducer of fevers. Some Hill Tribes use the flowers in the steam bath or sauna to treat vertigo, low energy, and fainting, and as a general tonic for health and longevity.

This is the national tree and national flower of Thailand.

· · · · ·

GREEN TEA
Camelia sinensis
chaa kǐeow | cha khiao
ชาเขียว

TASTE: *Astringent*
PART USED: *Leaves*

Internal Application: Green tea's beneficial properties are due to tannins, natural antibiotic compounds that occur naturally in the leaf. In modern times, green tea has been shown to be rich in antioxidants, which seems to confirm its long-standing reputation as a general tonic. Taken regularly, green tea promotes a healthy immune system, protecting against infections and cancers of the respiratory and digestive systems.

Green tea has a regulating and alkalizing effect on the digestive system, and helps both constipation and diarrhea. In general, it is useful as a digestive, although different processing and roasting methods produce differing results. Green tea also is beneficial for blood circulation, aids in disinfecting bacterial infections of the mouth, and protects against tooth and gum disease.

External Application: Green tea leaves can be used to treat wounds; however, there are better herbs for this purpose.

· · · · ·

GUAVA
Psidium guajava
fà-ràng | farang
ฝรั่ง

TASTE: *Astringent*
PART USED: *Leaf, fruit*

Internal Application: Guava leaves treat diarrhea if caused by excess Water Element, as well as stomachache and peptic ulcers. They are also beneficial for the immune system. Guava tea treats blocked or irregular menstruation and cases of chronic stress or anxiety.

External Application: Guava leaves get rid of bad smells and some skin fungi; however, they are not often used for external medicine.

Derived from the Thai word for "French," farang translates literally as "foreigner," and specifically connotes a Western foreigner. As you might suspect from this, guavas are not native to Thailand. They were introduced by the Portuguese approximately 400 years ago and have existed in Thailand long enough to become a part of the medicinal repertoire.

· · · · ·

GUDUCHI
Tinospora crispa
bor rá pét | boraphet
บอระเพ็ด

TASTE: *Bitter, Cooling*
PART USED: *Stem*

Internal Application: Guduchi is beneficial for the liver and the blood. It treats fever, stimulates the appetite, and expels intestinal parasites. It is used for stomach problems in babies, malaria, eye and ear diseases, and mucus congestion. Guduchi also beneficial for those with diabetes.

. . . . .

HARITAKI
Terminalia chebula
sà-mŏr-tai | samo thai
สมอไทย

TASTE: *Astringent, Sour, Bitter*
PART USED: *Fruit*

Internal Application: The unripe fruit is a common detoxifying remedy for fever, parasitic infections, spleen disorders, jaundice, skin disease, and allergic reactions of the skin. Haritaki corrects digestive disorders, and can be used for constipation, diarrhea, dysentery, and other intestinal parasites.

It also has a beneficial effect on the nervous system, nervous disorders, and cancerous tumors. It is an expectorant used for colds, congestion, cough, asthma, bronchitis, and laryngitis, and an astringent used to halt mucus or blood in the stool, sputum, or vaginal discharge. The ripe fruit has an astringent and antidiarrheal effect. Haritaki balances the Elements and rejuvenates the body and mind. It also expels toxins and promotes bowel movements.

External Application: Fresh haritaki can be used to make an infusion for use as an eye wash for injured eyes.

Haritaki holds a special place in Buddhism around Asia. The Medicine Buddha, one of the chief Buddhist deities in East Asian and Tibetan Buddhism, is commonly depicted holding a haritaki fruit in his hand. It is also found in the ancient Ayurvedic formula triphala, used across Asia.

. . . . .

HANUMAN PRASAN KAI
Schefflera leucantha
hà-nú-maan bprà-săan gaai | hanuman prasan kai
หนุมานประสานกาย

TASTE: *Spicy/Hot, Bitter, Astringent*
PART USED: *Whole plant*

Internal Application: Hanuman prasan kai is used extensively to treat asthma and other upper respiratory ailments, including cough, bronchitis, colds, and respiratory tract infections. It is also beneficial for the promotion of circulation.

External Application: The leaves of this herb are beneficial for healing wounds, treating contusions, and stopping bleeding. It is also used in herbal mosquito repellents.

There is no Western common name for this herb, hence only the Thai and botanical names are given. Hanuman prasan krai can be purchased in the West online, where it is generally sold as an anti-asthmatic herbal supplement.

． ． ． ． ．

HENNA
Lawsonia inermis
tian ging | tian king
เทียนกิ่ง

TASTE: *Astringent, Pra (an unpleasant taste)*
PART USED: *Leaf*

External Application: The fresh henna leaf may be applied as a topical antiseptic to fungal and/or bacterial infections of the skin and nails. It is also used to treat ringworm, and may be used orally as a gargle for mouth and gum disease or infections.

． ． ． ． ．

HONEY
Excretions of the honey bee (Apis spp.)
nám pêung | nam phueng
น้ำผึ้ง

TASTE: *Sweet, Astringent, slightly Heating*

Internal Application: Honey is said to be "scraping," meaning that it has the ability to cut through and dissolve mucus. It is therefore extremely beneficial for sore throats with mucus, as well as other upper respiratory mucus-related ailments, such as asthma and cough. Honey is rejuvenating and increases vitality. It is beneficial for weak and depleted people, restorative to men who have recently ejaculated (which in Thai medicine is considered to be a loss of "essence"), and nourishes women who are menstruating. Honey is found as an adjuvant in many internal formulas as it assists in moving the herbs to the tissue.

External Application: Honey soothes and heals wounds, and is a natural antibacterial agent.

While all sugars are cooling, honey is the warmest sweetener there is, and is therefore the best sweetener for people with Water as their core Elemental constitution, or agitated Water Element. Honey is one of the five foods that the Buddha is said to have specifically recommended as medicine in the Theravada Buddhist monastic code.

The Thai word for honey translates as "bee water." In Thailand, it is very common to find honey that is wildcrafted, gathered from wild bee trees, and often comes with honeycombs and bee larvae for added nutritional benefit. Honey is considered a rather magical substance due to its connections with the Bud-

dha's teachings, its ability to transport herbs to the tissues, and its inability to be replaced by any other herb. For medicines that call for honey, there is no substitute.

. . . . .

IVY GOURD
Coccinia grandis
dtam-leung | tamlueng
ตำลึง

TASTE: *Cooling*
PART USED: *Leaves, stem*

Internal Application: Ivy gourd is a vine used as a purgative and for food poisoning. It treats fever and is used by some Hill Tribes as a tonic.

External Application: The juice from the leaves treats insect bites, burning pain, and eye conditions, such as redness and pain.

Ivy gourd can be added to any Thai curry recipe.

. . . . .

JACKFRUIT
Artocarpus heterophyllus
kà-nǔn | khanun
ขนุน

TASTE: *The fruit is Sweet. The leaf is Bitter. The seed is Oily.*
PART USED: *Fruit, leaf, seed*

Internal Application: The leaf of the jackfruit is beneficial for blood, treats venereal diseases, and calms the nerves. The seed aids milk production and promotes milk flow. It also gives energy. All over Thailand, the fleshy tulip-shaped segments of the fruit are eaten raw when ripe, and are cooked in curries when unripe. The seeds are boiled or roasted and are eaten in curry. As it is a nutritive tonic high in caloric energy, jackfruit seed is especially useful in convalescence, in cases of low immunity, low energy, chronic fatigue, or chronic illness, and in old age. Decoction of the root is used to treat diarrhea.

The jackfruit is an enormous fruit, which often grows up to 3 feet in length. The heartwood of the jackfruit tree is used by monks in rural northeastern Thailand's Forest Tradition monasteries to dye their robes. Chips of wood are boiled in water, producing a rich dye called gaen-kanun, which is held to have remarkable medicinal qualities. In fact, monks of this tradition never wash their robes. Once a week, the robes are reboiled in jackfruit dye and are hung to dry in the sun. Robes treated in this manner are said to never smell bad, and monks swear by the protection the dyed robes impart to the skin—such as immunity from fungal infections, skin disorders, and disagreeable body odor.

. . . . .

JASMINE
Jasminum spp.
má-lí | mali
มะลิ

TASTE: *Fragrant/Cool, Bitter*
PART USED: *Flower*

Internal Application: In TTM texts, jasmine is said to be beneficial for calming the heart-mind and easing anxiety. It decreases toxins resulting from excess heat, treats fever, and eases excessive thirst from fever. Jasmine is also a heart tonic, and is beneficial for the fetus. It alleviates pain in the eyes as well.

External Application: Jasmine is used in steams and herbal compresses prepared by traditional medicine practitioners. It is also infused into oils and added to incense to ease the heart-mind and relieve anxiety. It can also be added to herbal oils that are used for massage or applied to the body for this same purpose.

There are many species of jasmine that may be used medicinally, all of which are called má-lí. Here we are referring to the common jasmine. Dried jasmine of different varieties can be found in the West at Chinese herbal supply shops, online herbal suppliers, and local Western herb shops. Jasmine garlands are frequently used as offerings on Buddhist altars and in Buddhist temples throughout Thailand. They are also given as blessings to friends and family on certain holidays.

. . . . .

KAFFIR LIME
Citrus hystix
má grùut | makrut
มะกรูด

TASTE: *The fruit is Sour. The leaves are Fragrant/Cool.*
PART USED: *Fruit, leaves*

Internal Application: Taken internally, kaffir lime is a digestion stimulant that alleviates flatulence and indigestion and is used to promote regularity in the case of blocked or infrequent menstruation. It is well known as a blood purifier, as an antioxidant with cancer-preventing properties, and as a treatment for high blood pressure.

External Application: Used externally, kaffir lime is beneficial for its antiseptic and aromatic properties, as well as its ability to clear toxins from the blood. It is a tonic for the heart-mind, and is frequently found in hot herbal compresses as well as in Thai herbal balms and liniments. When used in compresses and herbal steams, the vapors are calming. It is also found in formulas for the scalp, hair, and skin.

Kaffir lime fruit, and more commonly, leaves, can be found in the West at many Asian food stores and some specialty markets. Live kaffir lime plants can be bought at nurseries as well, often grafted on to other citrus plants in order to endure a cooler climate.

· · · · ·

LACQUER TREE
Melanorrhoea usitata
rák yài | rak yai
รักใหญ่

TASTE: *Astringent*
PART USED: *Leaves*

Internal Application: Tea from the leaves of the lacquer tree is used traditionally to treat diarrhea and intestinal parasites such as dysentery.

External Application: A poultice can be made to apply topically for joint pains and arthritis.

The Thai name for the lacquer tree, rak yai, translates as "big love." While the poisonous sap is no longer used for lacquer, the trees do continue to be used for wood and are the source of a dark dye used traditionally for dying robes and for ink.

· · · · ·

LEMONGRASS
Cymbopogon citratus
dtà-krái | takhrai
ตะไคร้

TASTE: *Aromatic Pungent*
PART USED: *Lower half of stalk*

Internal Application: Lemongrass tea is used as a therapy for colds (especially colds with fever), congestion, cough, sore throat, and laryngitis. Lemongrass is useful as a digestion stimulant in cases of flatulence, indigestion, and constipation. It is also used to counter stomach pains, nausea, vomiting, and back pain, as well as being a diuretic. Lemongrass is used by some Hill Tribes as a general tonic, for bone and joint pain. Lemongrass tea soothes menstrual pain.

External Application: Lemongrass vapors, from hot herbal compresses, herbal steams, and inhalation of herbal balms and liniments, are calming to the heart-mind and relieve stress. Lemongrass in external herbal products aids in dispersing stagnation and moves the blood. It can be used in balms to sooth menstrual pain but is stronger when taken internally. Topically, lemongrass destroys bacteria and fungi.

In Thailand, it is common to give babies a stalk of lemongrass to chew on when they are teething. Citronella grass, known in Thailand as ta krai hom ตะไคร้หอม, is closely related to lemongrass. Citronella, however, is primarily used as an insect repellent and is not used as an internal medicine.

. . . . .

LICORICE
Glycyrrhiza glabra
Chá aym tâyt | Cha-em thet
ชะเอมเทศ

TASTE: *Sweet*
PART USED: *Root*

Internal Application: Licorice root is most commonly used in the Thai tradition as a cold remedy, as well as for flu, cough, congestion, and fever. It is useful for soothing mucus membranes, and may be used in cases of stomach pain, peptic ulcers, sore throat, laryngitis, lung disease, and bronchial infections. Licorice is an expectorant, hence it moves mucus. Licorice is frequently found in herbal tea pills formulated for cough. Licorice clears toxins from the blood and is beneficial for the mind.

External Application: Licorice can be found in various topical formulas, including compresses, balms, and liniments.

. . . . .

LIME
Citrus aurantifolia
má naao | manao
มะนาว

TASTE: *Sour*
PART USED: *Fruit*

Internal Application: The fruit of the lime cuts through mucus, and clears the mucus membrane. The juice of the fruit is used as a vehicle to activate the properties of other medicines. This is why many medicinal formulas must be taken with lime juice.

External Application: Topically, lime treats poisonous bites, calms the mind, opens the nasal passages, and treats the tissue level of the body.

The Thai language uses the same word for both lemons and limes. Lemons are extremely rare in Thailand, though. So, while it is common for English menus in Thailand to list "lemonade," what you are most likely to be served is limeade.

· · · · ·

LONG PEPPER
Piper longum
dee bplee | di pli
ดีปลี

TASTE: *Spicy/Hot, Bitter*
PART USED: *Fruit*

Internal Application: Long pepper regulates and promotes the menses, builds blood, moves clots, and circulates blood. It is also an expectorant that moves congestion and treats cold, wet ailments. Long pepper is found in many Thai herbal formulas

External Application: Long pepper is used in external formulas to move the blood and reduce pain.

Long pepper is the principal herb associated with the Element Earth and is found in the Benjagoon formula for this reason. When buying long pepper in the West, make sure that it is about 1 inch long and at least ¼-inch thick. We have found that the long pepper sold in the West is frequently much too small. Whether this is the immature Piper longum or another plant altogether, it is not an adequate replacement.

C A U T I O N: Use of long pepper is contraindicated during pregnancy, as the same ability to move blood and clots can cause miscarriage.

· · · · ·

LONGAN
Dimocarpus longan
lam yai | lamyai
ลำไย

TASTE: *Sweet*
PART USED: *Fruit*

Internal Application: Longan fruit is eaten extensively in Thailand, especially in the north, where it is widely cultivated. Both the fruit and the tea made from the bark are said to relieve digestive discomfort, and the dried fruit is said to reduce fever. Longan fruit, often called "longan berries," is considered to be a nutritive tonic, good for people in weakened or depleted states.

Longan is used medicinally throughout Southeast Asia and China. In Thailand, it is primarily the fruit that is utilized, but, in other countries, the seeds and roots are also thought to have medicinal value. The dried fruit is sold as a snack food throughout Thailand.

Both fresh and dried longan fruit are sold in Western Asian food markets, and the dried fruit can be found in Chinese herb shops.

· · · · ·

LOTUS
Nelumbo nucifera
bua-lŭang | bua luang
บัวหลวง

TASTE: *The flower and stamens are Astringent and Fragrant/Cool. The seeds are Oily.*
PART USED: *Flower, stamen, seed*

Internal Application: The seed of the lotus is used in Thai medicine as a general nutritive tonic, especially during pregnancy. As part of the daily diet, the seeds are beneficial for skin, bones, muscles, and joints. Lotus seed is a cardiac tonic recommended to strengthen the heart muscle. Inhaled, the vapor of the flower calms the heart-mind, promoting a clear and peaceful mental state. Lotus stamen may also be taken internally as a remedy for dizziness and nervousness.

External Application: Lotus flowers are occasionally used in hot herbal compresses formulated for prenatal work, as they are calming and soothing to the fetus.

The lotus is revered across Asia wherever Hinduism and Buddhism predominate, and it is the most sacred plant in Thailand. Lotus flowers can be found growing on the grounds of most temples, and many universities and government buildings. They are commonly given to monks by the devout as symbols of reverence, and are positioned prominently upon Buddhist altars across the country. The lotus is symbolic of the human soul's transmigration through life. Growing in swamps, the plant begins its life cycle under muddy water, slowly breaking through to the surface, where it blooms. Similarly, in the Buddhist and Hindu belief system, the individual is reincarnated again and again in the "mud" of the world, until it breaks through to the surface and blooms in enlightenment.

Lotus seeds can be purchased in the West in Asian food markets.

· · · · ·

MACE
Myristica fragrans
dòk-jan | dokchan
ดอกจันทน์

TASTE: *Spicy/Hot*
PART USED: *The aril (covering) of the nutmeg seed*

Internal Application: Mace is calming to the heart-mind and the Subtle Winds. It is also a blood tonic.

External Application: Mace is also used in topical liniments and other formulas for the same purposes as its internal application.

Mace comes from the same plant as nutmeg, and therefore they share a botanical name. The decision to present them separately in this compendium was based on the fact that they are treated as separate herbs in Thai herbal medicine.

· · · · ·

MANGO
Mangifera india
má-mûang | mamuang
มะม่วง

TASTE: *Unripe mango is Astringent and Sour. Ripe mango is Sweet and Heating.*
PART USED: *Fruit*

Internal Application: The sour young fruit dissolves phlegm. Mango is a blood purifier and is beneficial for those who live in highly polluted areas. It is recommended for the elderly, and for those experiencing chronic illness.

There are many varieties of mango in Thailand, which are eaten both ripe and unripe. The unripe mango is tart and crunchy, and often pickled and/or served with a dip made of sugar, salt, and chilies. Mango is high in vitamin C.

· · · · ·

MANGOSTEEN
Garcinia mangostana
mang kút | mangkhut
มังคุด

TASTE: *The rind is Astringent. The fruit is Cooling and Sweet.*
PART USED: *Rind, fruit*

Internal Application: The rind of the mangosteen is beneficial for diarrhea caused by excess Water Element, dysentery, and hemorrhoids. Mangosteen is known to boost immunity, prevent cancer, and promote general health. Powder from the rind is also traditionally used to counter food poisoning, food allergies, and arthritis.

External Application: The rind is used topically as an astringent poultice to cleanse cuts, wounds, and skin infections.

Mangosteen has gained fame in the West in recent years as a superfood capable of providing incredible health benefits. In Thailand, it is known as the Queen of Fruits, as the inner flesh is one of the sweetest fruits known, and it is very cooling. Mangosteen season coincides nicely with durian season, and the two fruits are often paired as the King and Queen of Fruits. (Durian is very Spicy/Hot, and one of the most heating fruits there is.)

Mangosteens are eaten raw, but only the white inner section is consumed. Or, you can juice them—skin and all—for maximum nutritional benefit. When shopping for mangosteens, look for fruits with no cracks or yellow resin. Count the leaves on the cap (the more the better), as more leaves means more sections inside, and more sections means fewer large, bitter seeds.

· · · · ·

MARIJUANA
Cannibis sativa
gan chaa | kancha
กัญชา

TASTE: *Toxic*
PART USED: *Whole plant*

Internal Application: Marijuana traditionally treats insomnia, and is used in cases of wasting diseases because it stimulates the appetite. It is also used for pain control.

External Application: Externally, marijuana seeds are an ingredient in traditional analgesic liniments for pain.

The Thai name clearly comes from the Sanskrit word ganja, variations of which are found globally. A fun side note is that the Thai word for catnip, gan chaa maew กัญชาแมว, translates as "ganja for cats."

C A U T I O N: Marijuana is contraindicated for postpartum nursing mothers, as it has been shown to decrease lactation. Being fat soluble, the drug also enters the milk in low doses and is passed on to the infant. Medicinally, marijuana is best ingested through teas, powders, and other orally ingested formulas as the smoke commonly used for recreational use is carcinogenic.

· · · · ·

MENTHOL
Mentha spp.
grèt sà-rá-nàe | kret saranae
เกร็ดสะระแหน่

TASTE: *Fragrant/Cool*
PART USED: *Crystals derived from the mint plant*

Internal Application: Treats nausea, indigestion, sore throats, and headache, as well as asthma and bronchitis.

External Application: Menthol is a common ingredient in Thai herbal balms and liniments formulated to cool inflammation and treat acute injury. In addition to cooling, menthol has a slight numbing effect on pain. Mentholated balms and liniments are applied topically to the temples for headache and to relieve itching.

· · · · ·

MILK
nom | nom
นม

TASTE: *Sweet, Oily*
PART USED: *Milk from cows or goats*

Internal Application: Milk is a nutritive tonic, and may be used in preparations to counter low energy, low immunity, emaciation, and to build strength in children, the elderly, and those convalescing from disease or injury.

External Application: Milk soothes rashes, chemical burns, and many allergic skin reactions. Powdered milk is beneficial as a topical treatment for dry or scaly skin.

While many people in the world, especially in Asia, are lactose intolerant, the medicinal use of milk is part of traditional healing arts. For those who abstain from milk for religious, ethical, physical, or spiritual reasons, almond milk is the plant-based milk with properties closest to mammal milk. However, it must be home made in order to be medicinally used, as the mass-produced versions currently available at the grocery store are mostly water with thickeners. See note about milk on page 37.

C A U T I O N: Milk should not be used for illnesses with excessive congestion, as it thickens mucus.

· · · · ·

MINT
Mentha spp.
sà-rá-nàe | saranae
สะระแหน่

TASTE: *Aromatic Pungent*
PART USED: *Leaves*

Internal Application: Peppermint tea is a general digestion stimulant, and is the preferred treatment for stomach spasms or pains, nausea, abdominal cramps, indigestion, irritable bowel syndrome, and gastritis. Tea or inhalation of mint vapor is prescribed to treat cough. Peppermint has a calming effect on the heart-mind, and the vapor is used with success in the treatment of nervousness, insomnia, and stress-related or migraine headaches.

External Application: In topical formulas, mint relieves inflammation and cools the skin.

Mint has the dual ability to be either heating or cooling. If taken internally it is more heating, whereas it is more cooling when used topically. There are many types of mint, including peppermint, spearmint, and mountain mint, which can all be used in formulas requiring mint. The three just listed are ordered from mildest to strongest.

· · · · ·

MORINGA [HORSERADISH TREE]
Moringa oleifera
má rum | marum
มะรุม

TASTE: *The fruit is Heating. The bark is Chum. The seeds are Tasteless and Oily.*
The root is Spicy/Hot, Sweet, and Bitter.
PART USED: *Whole plant*

Internal Application: Moringa fruit is beneficial as a cardiac tonic and to prevent fainting. Decoction of the bark is a digestion stimulant used traditionally for combating flatulence, indigestion, and bloated stomach.

External Application: Decoction of the root is a disinfectant, and may be used as an astringent to stop bleeding and help promote the healing of wounds. The seeds, when roasted and ground, are made into a poultice for arthritis.

In Thailand, moringa has been called a wonder tree for its ability to assist life and health. Some global health organizations use it to maintain nutrition levels in malnourished populations. Chum is an untranslatable word indicating a strong "funky" taste that is often perceived as unpleasant. It is often musky, or pungent and odiferous.

· · · · ·

MORNING GLORY
[WATER SPINACH, WATER MORNING GLORY]
Ipomoea aquatica
pàk-bûng | phak bung
ผักบุ้ง

TASTE: *Tasteless*
PART USED: *Stem, leaves*

Internal Application: Morning glory draws out poison and is used to make a detoxifying drink. It treats constipation, gonorrhea, nerves, insomnia, and blood in the feces. Morning glory also promotes good eyesight.

External Application: Externally, morning glory treats the eyes and abscesses.

NOTE: In the West, the common name "morning glory" is used for many plants, especially in the Convolvulaceae family. Here, we are referring to a different plant altogether, that is commonly sold under the name "morning glory" at Thai restaurants and Asian groceries.

· · · · ·

MOUSE PEPPER
Capiscum frutescens
prík-kêe-nŭu | phrik khi nu
พริกขี้หนู

TASTE: *Spicy/Hot, Heating*
PART USED: *Fruit*

Internal Application: Internally, chilies excite the Wind and can be used to treat cases of constipation caused by lack of digestive tract Wind. Also useful in cases of colds and congestion, chilies increase circulation and increase appetite. They can also treat flatulence.

External Application: Topically, chilies move blood and treat pain. They are a common ingredient in heating balms and liniments, although use caution to avoid irritating sensitive skin.

The Thai name for these peppers literally translates to "mouse shit pepper," referring to their shape and small size. While Thai cuisine uses both green and red chilies, for medicinal purposes it is best to use the more mature red ones.

· · · · ·

MULBERRY
Morus alba
dtôn mòn | ton mon
ต้นหม่อน

TASTE: *The fruit is Sour, Sweet, and Cooling. The leaves are Cooling. The bark is Tasteless.*
PART USED: *Leaves, fruit, root*

Internal Application: The leaves and fruit relieve fever and thirst as well as cough. The leaves treat eye disorders including conjunctivitis. Mulberry leaves are diuretic as well as beneficial for reducing blood pressure. The fruit is beneficial for the kidneys, loosens bowels, and treats rheumatism. Mulberry root has been shown to have tumor-shrinking properties. In larger doses, mulberry is used as a purgative to expel tapeworms and other intestinal parasites. Its leaves treat indigestion and flatulence as well as diarrhea.

External Application: The leaves are beneficial for the skin.

· · · · ·

MYRRH
Commiphora myrrha
gam-yaan | kamyan
กำยาน

TASTE: *Astringent, Fragrant/Cool*
PART USED: *Resin from tree*

Internal Application: Myrrh treats uterine bleeding, arthritis, circulatory problems, and pain.

External Application: Myrrh is drawing and antifungal. It disperses blood, lowers inflammation, and reduces pain. It is found in liniments for acute injuries.

· · · · ·

NEEM

Azadirachta indica
sà-dao | sadao
สะเดา

TASTE: *Bitter*
PART USED: *Whole plant*

Internal Application: Neem leaf and wood prevent fever and balance the Elements. They also stimulate the appetite. The bark of the stem is used as an astringent to treat dysentery and diarrhea. The root is used as an expectorant, a bitter tonic and an antimalarial. The heartwood effectively treats nausea, vomit, and parasites, and is used to calm chronic anxiety and stress, as well as delirium due to high fever.

The fruit is an anthelmintic, meaning that it contains a substance that purges intestinal parasites, and is also an astringent for hemorrhoids and a treatment for malaria. The young shoots, leaves, and flowers are used as a bitter tonic for detoxification of blood, as well as for treatment of vomiting, stomach pain, indigestion, fever, and malaria. Decoction of these parts is also a general internal antibacterial, antiviral, and diuretic used frequently to treat dysentery, diarrhea, and parasites. Chewing the stems is said to stimulate the appetite. The Wat Pho texts mention the seed as a mild stimulant and as a treatment for poisoning.

External Application: The young stems of the neem tree are used throughout South Asia as a toothbrush. The ends of the stem are chewed until fine and stringy, and are then rubbed against the teeth and gums to cleanse and stimulate. Neem oil is used in natural toothpaste preparations throughout South Asia, and may also be used as a mouthwash or gargle on a daily basis. It is an antiseptic for mouth sores, gum disease, oral infections, and abscesses. Due to its antibacterial properties, the oil of the neem tree is a common additive to soap and shampoo, and may also be dropped into the ear canal to treat infections.

Applied to the skin, the leaf, seed, and/or oil treat fungal infections, eczema, acne, scabies, lice, ringworm, and other skin parasites, and may safely be used as a vaginal douche for infections. Some Hill Tribes use neem for dermatitis, rash, and warts. Neem oil is often used in cosmetic skin preparations to enhance skin tone, elasticity, and youthfulness. It is also an effective insecticide.

· · · · ·

NONI [INDIAN MULBERRY]
Morinda citrifolia
yor | yo
ยอ

TASTE: *Heating*
PART USED: *Fruit*

Internal Application: In TTM, noni is used to relieve muscle pain and vomiting, and to reduce blood pressure. It is also used as a digestive, and to treat nausea and vomiting. Noni is beneficial for colds, tuberculosis, flu, parasites, and gastritis. In modern Thailand, it is used as a daily tonic in the treatment of cancer, HIV/AIDS, hepatitis, and other severe diseases.

· · · · ·

NUTGRASS
Cyperus rotundus
hâew mǒo | haeo mu
แห้วหมู

TASTE: *Aromatic Pungent*
PART USED: *Rhizome*

Internal Application: Taken daily, nutgrass is a tonic for the liver and heart, a stimulant for digestion, and an aid against hypertension. It is extremely useful in cases of blocked or infrequent menstruation, menstrual cramps, and PMS. In Thai tradition, it is used to treat fevers, especially those that occur during menstruation. It is also commonly used to treat diarrhea, dysentery, stomach or intestinal cramps, irritable bowel, gastritis indigestion, flatulence, colds, flu, and congestion.

· · · · ·

NUTMEG
Myristica fragrans
lùuk jan | luk chan
ลูกจันทน์

TASTE: *Aromatic Pungent, slightly Astringent*
PART USED: *Wood, seed*

Internal Application: Nutmeg is beneficial for the heart and helps to flush blood throughout the body. Nutmeg calms the nerves, mind, and Subtle Winds. The seed kernel is properly called nutmeg, while the membrane that covers the kernel is called mace. Nutmeg is used in small quantities in Thai cuisine as an appetizer, digestive, and carminative. It is added as a spice to food to enhance assimilation of food, lessen flatulence, and correct sluggish digestion. Nutmeg is also considered to be a tonic for the blood and a sedative with muscle-relaxing qualities.

External Application: Nutmeg is beneficial when incorporated into oils used topically to soothe the heart-mind and calm the Subtle Winds. It is also calming to the nerves.

Nutmeg comes from the same plant as mace, and therefore they share a botanical name. The decision to present them separately in this compendium was based on the fact that they are treated as separate herbs in Thai herbal medicine.

C A U T I O N: Nutmeg is toxic in high doses.

· · · · ·

ONION
Allium cepa
hŏm | hom
หอม

TASTE: *Spicy/Hot*
PART USED: *Bulb*

Internal Application: Onions are beneficial for treating colds, cough, and upper respiratory ailments.

External Application: Onions are drawing, and are therefore found in poultices and hot herbal compresses formulated to draw out toxins. They can be used for treatment of warts. Onion vapors are used to treat colds in children.

C A U T I O N: Note that it is important to use an onion that is freshly cut—not one that was previously cut and left out or refrigerated.

· · · · ·

OPIUM POPPY
Papaver somniferum
dtôn fìn | ton fin
ต้นฝิ่น

TASTE: *Toxic*
PART USED: *Flowers, seeds, sap*

Internal Application: While opium addiction and narcotics trafficking are two of Thailand's most pressing social problems, the opium poppy has long been esteemed by traditional herbalists for its potent effects. Taken internally, opium is one of the most effective natural anesthetics, and it is traditionally employed to these purposes in rural Thailand, where modern anesthetics are unavailable. In small doses, opium is a mild stimulant. In larger doses, it is used as a temporary calmative in severe cases of anxiety, stress, or panic attacks. The seeds of the poppy, commonly available commercially, have an astringent effect, and are taken to treat diarrhea and dysentery. Opium is additionally mentioned in the Wat Pho texts as an effective remedy for cough, rectal bleeding, and hemorrhoids.

External Application: A poultice of opium resin is used topically as a local analgesic for management of pain and soothing of muscle spasms. It may be applied to the temples to alleviate headache.

In most countries, opium itself is illegal, but opium poppies are often legal as ornamental flowers. Given the widespread abuse and social problems associated with opium, as well as its illegal status in most countries, the authors do not condone its use. We provide information on the traditional use of this plant only as a point of cultural interest.

· · · · ·

OTAHEITE GOOSEBERRY
Phyllanthus acidus
má yom | mayom
มะยม

TASTE: *Sour*
PART USED: *Fruit*

Internal Application: Otaheite gooseberries are a blood tonic. They are also a laxative, and are used to move phlegm and relieve cough. Otaheite gooseberries are traditionally eaten to alleviate cases of fever, chronic thirst, and measles, and are general immunity boosters.

· · · · ·

OYSTER SHELL
hǒi naang rom | hoi nangrom
หอยนางรม

TASTE: *Salty*

Internal Application: Ground oyster shells are a traditional treatment for kidney stones, flatulence, and indigestion. Due to the high calcium content of the shell, it is also recommended as a dietary supplement for those with bone disease or fractures.

· · · · ·

PALM SUGAR
Borassus flabellifer
nám-dtaan bpèuk | namtan puek
น้ำตาลปึก

TASTE: *Sweet*
PART USED: *Sap*

Internal Application: Palm sugar is highly nutritive, so it is beneficial for cases of depletion and weakness. It is beneficial for children, supports the Water Element, and is both hydrating and strengthening. Palm sugar is used extensively in Thailand as a natural sweetener that does not spike blood sugar levels as white sugar does. Minimally processed, it retains its nutrient value and is an excellent alternative to other sweeteners.

Palm sugar should not be confused with coconut sugar. Palm sugar comes from the sap of a variety of sugar palms, and, when purchased through Asian food markets, is remarkably less expensive than other natural sweeteners.

Palm sugar is commonly sold in hard discs or spires. Look for the less-processed tan-colored palm sugar, and avoid it if it is white. To make syrup, place the disc in a pot and fill with water to about twice its height. Heat slowly over very low heat until dissolved, then store in a jar. For thicker syrup, use less water. A similar sugar, also made from sugar palms, is jaggery. Used widely in India, this is palm sugar as well, but it is processed differently resulting in a darker color and stronger taste.

· · · · ·

PANDANUS [PANDAN LEAVES]
Pandanus amaryllifolius
bai dtoie | bai toei
ใบเตย

TASTE: *Sweet, Fragrant/Cool*
PART USED: *Leaves*

Internal Application: Pandanus is beneficial for the heart, lowers cholesterol levels, and is known as a pain reliever. The leaves are chewed for oral pain, and are used for easing stomach cramping. Pandanus also reduces fever and mucus congestion, and relieves indigestion and flatulence.

External Application: Pandanus leaves are beneficial for wounds, and bathing in water with pandanus leaf juice eases sunburn.

Pandanus is used extensively in Thai cooking as both a flavoring and coloring agent. The juice from the leaves is found in both sweet and savory dishes, and is used perhaps in an analogous way to how Western cooking uses vanilla. Pandanus leaves are also frequently mixed with other herbs to make tea.

· · · · ·

PAPAYA
Carica papaya
má lá gor | malako
มะละกอ

TASTE: *The unripe fruit is Sour. The ripe fruit is Sweet. The seed is Bitter and Astringent.*
PARTS USED: *Fruit, seed*

Internal Application: The unripe papaya fruit is a digestive; the ripe fruit and the seeds are mild laxatives taken medicinally to treat constipation, indigestion, flatulence, and cramping of the intestines. Papaya seed is also used to purge dysentery and other parasites of the gastrointestinal tract, as well as to treat ringworm. The root is a diuretic used to treat venereal diseases such as gonorrhea, and the stem treats leucorrhea. Papaya is recommended as part of the daily diet for cases of arthritis, allergies, asthma, hypertension, influenza, toothaches, and cancerous tumors. Either the seeds or the fruit may be taken as a general tonic for low immunity, low energy, chronic fatigue, and wasting diseases.

External Application: The leaf of the papaya is used topically on wounds, skin ulcers, and other sores as it cleanses and speeds healing.

Papaya stimulates and aids digestion due to the large amount of the papain enzyme present in the fruit. The juice or fruit can also can be used as a marinade to tenderize tough meat for the same reason. Papaya also contains large quantities of vitamins A and C, well-known antioxidants. The fruit of the papaya is eaten both ripe and unripe (see Chapter 3 for a recipe based on unripe papaya).

· · · · ·

PARACRESS
Acmella oleracea
pàk krâat hŭa waen | phak khrat hua waen
ผักคราดหัวแหวน

TASTE: *Slightly Toxic*
PART USED: *Whole plant*

Internal Application: Paracress tea is a digestion stimulant. It is useful in cases of flatulence, nausea, and vomiting, and is also prescribed for fever, arthritis, and gout. Mixed with vinegar, it makes a mild antiseptic for mouth sores and sore throat. The stems are also chewed for toothaches, and are sometimes given to children with speech disorders or stutters. Paracress is said to cure these problems.

- - - - -

PINEAPPLE
Ananas comosus
sàp-bpà-rót | sapparot
สับปะรด

TASTE: *The fruit is Sweet and Sour. The rhizome is Sweet and Cooling.*
PART USED: *Fruit, rhizome*

Internal Application: The rhizome of the pineapple plant is a diuretic recommended for those suffering from kidney diseases, kidney stones, bladder infections, and urinary tract infections. Pineapple fruit juice is recommended for inflammatory internal diseases, diseases of the liver, and cough or cold with congestion. It is a nutritive tonic for convalescents, and is said to detoxify the entire system. It is also recommended for diseases of the uterus, for postpartum tonification, and for strengthening the female reproductive organs. The fruit juice is used in treatment of depression and is said to have an especially beneficial effect on the brain and nervous system. Some Hill Tribes use pineapple juice to treat stomachache.

External Application: Topically used on warts, rashes, and dermatitis.

- - - - -

PLANTAIN
Plantago spp.
yaa en yêut | ya en yuet
ยาเอ็นยืด

TASTE: *Sweet, Cooling*
PART USED: *Whole plant*

Internal Application: The plantain noted here is not to be confused with starchy bananas, also called plantain, which are a completely different plant. The fresh juice from the whole plantain plant is drunk as a diuretic to treat bladder or urinary tract infections, gastric inflammation, and kidney stones. It is an expectorant that helps clear up cough, laryngitis, sore throat, and other respiratory problems. It soothes digestive ailments, peptic ulcers, and gastritis. It is astringent, and can be used to counter mucus or blood in the stool, sputum, or vaginal discharge.

External Application: Used topically in poultices, balms, liniments, and creams, plantain has a general drawing property and specifically can draw out poisons. It treats skin infections, such as staphylococcus and shingles. Plantain soothes itching, relieves inflammation, and is excellent for rashes, insect bites and other painful skin conditions. Plantain also softens the tissues and treats hemorrhoids.

With about 200 species of plantain, we have chosen to simply note the genus. Herbalists can use whatever species grows in their neck of the woods, as plantain is found nearly the world over. Yaa en yêut, translates as "medicine to stretch the sên." From this, we can see how this herb is of particular interest to Thai bodyworkers, who address the sên, specifically the tendons, ligaments, blood vessels, and nerves. The doctrine of signatures applies here, as the visibility of the vein in the leaves is notable in all varieties of plantain.

· · · · ·

PLUMBAGO
Plumbago spp.
jàyt moon plerng | chetta mun phloeng
เจตมูลเพลิง

TASTE: *Heating*
PART USED: *Whole plant*

Internal Application: Plumbago stimulates the Fire Element and warms the body. The root is used to stimulate digestion and is a diaphoretic, meaning that it induces perspiration. The root and/or bark of the plumbago may be used to treat cases of blocked or infrequent menstruation. It increases female fertility—although it may stimulate miscarriage and should never be taken during pregnancy. Plumbago is also used to detoxify the blood, and is prized by some Hill Tribes as a general longevity tonic. The root is used to treat hemorrhoids. The aerial parts of the plant are used in treatment of kidney disease, kidney cramps, and accompanying back pain.

· · · · ·

POMEGRANATE
Punica granatum
táp tim | thapthim
ทับทิม

TASTE: *The fruit is Sweet and Sour. The rind is Astringent. The root and bark are Toxic.*
PART USED: *Fruit, root, bark, seeds*

Internal Application: Fresh pomegranate juice can be used to lower the body's temperature in cases of fever. The rind of the pomegranate is a strong astringent used to treat diarrhea, dysentery, blood or mucus in the stool, and food poisoning. The bark of the root is effective in purging tapeworm and other intestinal parasites. The Wat Pho texts mention pomegranate flowers as a tonic to improve the quality of breast milk. The seeds are used in formulas for digestive troubles.

External Application: Fresh pomegranate juice may be used topically as an astringent and antifungal, or as a gargle for sore throat or mouth sores.

· · · · ·

POMELO
Citrus maxima
sôm oh | som o
ส้มโอ

TASTE: *Fragrant/Cool*
PART USED: *Rind*

Internal Application: The rind of the pomelo is used in internal medicine formulas, especially for the heart.

External Application: The rind of the pomelo is found in herbal compresses and herbal inhalers for the purpose of calming the mind and benefiting the heart.

Pomelo fruit is a wonderful treat that is readily available in any Thai market. It looks like an overgrown grapefruit, with thick pulp.

· · · · ·

PUMPKIN [KABOCHA]
Cucurbita maxima or Cucurbita moschata
fák tong | fakthong
ฟักทอง

TASTE: *Oily and Sweet*
PART USED: *Seeds, flesh*

Internal Application: Pumpkin seeds expel worms and increase urination. Recent studies in Thailand show that the seeds prevent formation of kidney stones. The orange flesh is nourishing to the tissues, is high in beta-carotene, and helps prevent cancer. It also nourishes eyesight. The root treats cough and toxins.

External Application: Pumpkin soothes inflammation and contusions.

· · · · ·

PURPLE ALLAMANDA [BLUE TRUMPET VINE]
Thunbergia laurifolia
raang jèut | rangchuet
รางจืด

TASTE: *Tasteless*
PART USED: *Whole plant*

Internal Application: In the Thai tradition, purple allamanda is most commonly used as a detoxifying agent. The leaves and stem purify the blood, and are therefore used as an antidote to all kinds of poisonous foods or chemicals. Some Hill Tribes prescribe it for poisonous snake or insect bites. Its detoxifying properties make it the preferred treatment for hangovers, and it is taken daily to counter the cirrhosis (inflammation of the liver) associated with alcoholism. Purple allamanda is useful in treating indigestion, flatulence, diarrhea, mucus or blood in the stool, and intestinal parasites. It is also prescribed as a remedy for fever, allergies, and asthma, and is recommended for diabetes and hypoglycemia as it reputedly controls blood sugar levels.

This plant is mentioned in the Wat Pho texts as a remedy for vomiting in infants, blocked or ir-regular menstruation, gonorrhea, sores on the tongue and mouth, as a diuretic, and as a poultice for burns. Purple allamanda has been found effective in countering minor allergic reactions and intoler-ances (such as to MSG, alcohol, and so on). Recent research at Chiang Mai University also shows it to be promising in assisting farmers who are exposed to high levels of herbicides and pesticides.

External Application: Topically, the whole plant is ground and used as a poultice for snake bites.

While not generally available in the West as an herbal medicine, purple allamanda is sold as an ornamen-tal plant, so those wishing to obtain it can do so relatively easily.

C A U T I O N: Purple allamanda, as an antidote to poisons, cleans the blood extremely effectively. Be-cause of this, it is contraindicated for people who take life-sustaining medications, as it will purify even that out of the blood.

· · · · ·

RAILROAD VINE
[GOAT'S FOOT CREEPER, BEACH MORNING GLORY]
Ipomoea pes-caprae
pàk-bûng-tá-lay | phak bungthale
ผักบุ้งทะเล

TASTE: *Cooling*
PART USED: *Leaves*

External Application: Railroad vine is applied topically to soothe insect bites, inflammation, allergic reactions, hives, and rashes. A poultice of railroad vine relieves the painful sting of jellyfish, or it can be mixed with vinegar for added effect.

Given that this herb grows on the beaches of Southern Thailand, its ability to relieve jellyfish stings is quite fortunate. This herb grows in many places around the world and can be wildcrafted.

• • • • •

RANGOON CREEPER
Quisqualis indica
lép meu naang | lepmuenang
เล็บมือนาง

TASTE: *The flowers are Fragrant/Cool. The leaves are Heating. The seeds are Oily and Toxic.*
PART USED: *Flowers, leaves, seeds*

Internal Application: Rangoon creeper is a purgative traditionally used to expel tapeworms and other intestinal parasites. It can be used for children, as it is not too strong.

External Application: Leaves are used topically for swelling and inflammation

C A U T I O N: *Take only with cold water, as warm water may cause nausea.*

• • • • •

RICE
Oryza sativa
kâao | khao
ข้าว

TASTE: *Sweet, Oily*
PART USED: *Seed*

Internal Application: Unbleached white rice is a gentle nourishing food, the primary component of meals in Thailand, as it is all over South and East Asia. Rice is nourishing to weak and depleted patients. It is easy to digest, and therefore gentle on the system when the digestive Fire is weak. Rice water slows diarrhea.

External Application: White sticky rice, which is drying and drawing, is used topically to cool inflammation and treat poison.

The Thai word for rice is synonymous with food in general, and a meal simply doesn't count as a meal if it does not have rice. The most common type of Thai rice is jasmine rice, which is native to the country.

Red rice and sticky rice are also very common. Brown rice is not considered a healthy choice in TTM, as it is hard to digest. Those wishing to combine the nutritional value of brown rice with the gentleness of white rice can turn to Thai red rice. However, for medicinal purposes, stick with unbleached white rice.

· · · · ·

ROSELLE
Hibiscus sabdariffa
grà jíap | krachiap
กระเจี๊ยบ

TASTE: *Sour*
PART USED: *Flower*

Internal Application: Roselle tea or juice is primarily prescribed as a diuretic for cases of gallstones, kidney stones, and urinary tract infections. It is additionally used to treat indigestion, flatulence, peptic ulcer, fever, cough, hypertension, kidney cramps, and back pain. It is high in calcium, and therefore is added to the daily diet to treat and prevent tooth and bone deterioration. Roselle flower is reputed to lower blood cholesterol. The seed is also a diuretic, and a tonic for the Four Elements. Roselle is also said to be beneficial for heart disease and lowering cholesterol.

· · · · ·

SAFFLOWER
Carthamus tinctorius
dòk kam fŏi | dok khamfoi
ดอกคำฝอย

TASTE: *Sweet, Heating*
PART USED: *Flower, seed*

Internal Application: Safflower is a blood tonic. Dried safflower is also a tonic for the heart, nervous, and circulatory system. Because of its beneficial effect on the circulation, it is used to treat cases of male sexual dysfunction and to encourage regularity in cases of blocked, irregular, or painful menstruation in women. The flower is used as a calmative in cases of stress, anxiety, and panic attacks. It is also an effective therapy for colds, arthritis, and constipation. The seed is a purgative and expectorant, and may also be used to encourage menstruation and to lower cholesterol.

External Application: In external balms and liniments, safflower is beneficial for the blood. It disperses and is especially good for contusions. Safflower breaks up clots and brings the bruise up from the deep layers of the tissue.

· · · · ·

SAFFRON

Crocus sativus

yâa fà-ràn | yafaran

หญ้าฝรั่น

TASTE: *Fragrant/Cool*

PART USED: *Stamen*

Internal Application: Saffron helps to build essence, or vitality, and is a tonic for the Water Element. It is also a heart and liver tonic.

External Application: Saffron can be used topically to treat skin issues. However, it is a very expensive herb, so it not generally preferred for this purpose.

C A U T I O N: In Thailand, travelers are often amazed at the incredibly inexpensive "saffron" they find sold on the streets at tourist markets, only to get home and discover their "saffron" to be ineffective in the kitchen. The reason? It is really safflower, which is a wonderful medicinal herb but a poor replacement for saffron in cooking.

· · · · ·

SAKAAN

Piper interruptum

sàkáan | sakhan

สะค้าน

TASTE: *Heating, Spicy/Hot*

PART USED: *Vine*

Internal Application: Sakaan is used to treat flatulence, asthma, fever, and many issues of Wind Element. It is found in the Ayurvedic formula trisan that balances the Water Element, as well as in the Benjagoon Element balancing formula.

We have not come across an English common name for this plant. It is likely that it cannot be found in the West, hence we have suggested alternatives in the formulas that use sakaan in this book. However, it is one of the primary herbs in TTM, and if you are traveling in Thailand you should pick some up at an herb shop.

· · · · ·

SANDALWOOD TREE
Santalum album
jan tâyt | chan thet
จันทน์เทศ

TASTE: *Bitter, Fragrant/Cool*
PART USED: *Wood*

Internal Application: Sandalwood is soothing to the nerves and is used in formulas that treat depression, Subtle Winds, and anxiety. Sandalwood is taken internally to treat fever and to detoxify the blood. It is used by some Hill Tribes to revive unconscious patients, and as a tonic.

External Application: Topically, also, sandalwood is beneficial for the mind-heart and for calming the Subtle Winds. It is infused in oils for topical use, or crushed with other herbs in hot herbal compresses. Sandalwood oil is a frequent ingredient in soaps, shampoos, and fragrances, all of which have a cooling effect on the body. Sandalwood may also be applied to dermatitis, herpes, infection, and inflammation of the skin.

C A U T I O N: Sandalwood trees are endangered in both Thailand and India, where they are often illegally poached from national forests. For this reason, only Australian sandalwood should be purchased, and even this should be used only as truly needed.

· · · · ·

SEA HOLLY
Acanthus ebracteatus
ngèuak bplaa mǒr | ngueak pla mo
เหงือกปลาหมอ

TASTE: *Salty, Heating*
PART USED: *Whole plant*

Internal Application: Sea holly is used as a longevity tonic. It is good for the lymphatic system, and it treats many associated disorders. Sea holly is also used in cancer treatment.

External Application: Sea holly is used topically to treat abscesses.

· · · · ·

SEA SALT
gleua sà-mùt | kluea samut
เกลือสมุทร

TASTE: *Salty*

Internal Application: Salt aids the body in absorbing and retaining water. It is beneficial for bone, and acts as a vehicle to transport other medicinal herbs to the right place in the body. Salt is also used to treat wounds in the mouth, nasal passages, and eyes. Salt assists in purging through its action as a laxative.

External Application: Used in topical formulas such as compresses, salt treats the level of the bone. However, it is dependent on other herbs to penetrate through the initial layers of the body. Salt retains heat, and in hot herbal compresses it assists in keeping the compress warm. Salt draws out excess moisture, and is beneficial for reducing postpartum water excess, edema, and other complications involving retained water. For postpartum women, salt compresses or clay pots with hot salt inside are placed on the abdomen. Salt is also used to clean the teeth.

Salt is associated with Fire and Water, so it has both a heating quality and a cooling quality. It heats, but not too much, and it cools, but not too much. Salt in Thailand is primarily harvested from the sea, although there are some salt mines as well. In Northern Thailand, there is a small village where the well-water is salty enough that salt can be harvested.

C A U T I O N: Use of hot salt compresses and clay pots is contraindicated in pregnancy as drawing out excess fluid, while desirable postpartum, can be harmful during pregnancy.

· · · · ·

SENNA
Cassia acutifolia
má-kǎam kàek | makham khaek
มะขามแขก

TASTE: *Sour, slightly Sweet*
PART USED: *Leaves, pods*

Internal Application: Tea made from senna pods is a strong and effective laxative for treatment of constipation. The leaves are somewhat more gentle, and tea from the leaves is traditionally used as a mild laxative for the elderly. In smaller doses, senna stimulates the liver and encourages the production of bile, thereby aiding digestion.

External Application: Decoction of senna pods is an antiseptic. Applied topically, it is used traditionally as a treatment for bacterial and fungal skin infections. As a gargle, it is used to treat infections of the mouth, including tooth and gum disease, and mouth sores.

C A U T I O N: If taking senna for constipation, it is important to know the cause of constipation. Does it come from lack of Wind (movement), or from the quality of the feces (too hard or too sticky)? Senna should only be used with the first condition. Taking senna with Aromatic Pungent herbs, such as cardamom, cinnamon, or cloves, will decrease the possibility of cramping.

· · · · ·

SESAME SEEDS
Sesamum indicum
ngaa | nga
งา

TASTE: *Oily, Sweet, Bitter*
PART USED: *Seed, oil*

Internal Application: In Thai medicine, sesame seeds are recommended dietary supplements for sufferers of joint problems, tooth decay, and bone weakness. Sesame promotes strength and increases body warmth, and is therefore a nutritive tonic when incorporated into the daily diet. Sesame seed is also taken in cases of cough, constipation, hemorrhoids, and painful or blocked menstruation.

External Application: Sesame oil is used extensively as a topical treatment for Wind imbalance. It is also used as a beneficial base for many balms and liniments.

C A U T I O N: When using sesame oil medicinally, be sure to get raw sesame oil. Many sesame oils sold in stores are toasted for flavor, but this denatures the medicinal quality.

· · · · ·

SHALLOT
Allium cepa var. aggregatum
hŏm daeng | hom daeng
หอมแดง

TASTE: *Heating*
PART USED: *Bulb*

Internal Application: Shallots treat colds, phlegm, and fevers from colds and prevent the flu.

External Application: Shallots are used in Thai hot herbal compresses and drawing poultices. On the skin they are slightly astringent.

Chopped shallot or white onion is often wrapped in muslin or cheesecloth and placed under a child's pillow so that they will inhale the vapors.

C A U T I O N: When shallots are used medicinally, in most cases you cannot substitute onion. Also note that it is important to use shallot that is freshly cut—not one that was previously cut and left out or refrigerated.

. . . . .

SICHUAN LOVAGE [SZECHUAN LOVAGE]
Ligusticum wallichii
got hǔa bua | kot hua bua
โกฐหัวบัว

TASTE: *Oily, Mild, Fragrant/Cool*
PART USED: *Rhizome*

Internal Application: Sichuan lovage is beneficial for the Wind that circulates throughout the body, as well as for treatment of abnormal growths. It also regulates menstruation.

External Application: Sichuan lovage is found in liniments that treat trauma, as it assists with circulation.

. . . . .

SNAKE GRASS
Clinacanthus nutans
pá-yaa yor | phaya yo
พญายอ

TASTE: *Tasteless, Cooling*
PART USED: *Leaves*

Internal Application: Snake grass is used internally to treat poison.

External Application: A tincture or ointment of snake grass is used topically to soothe skin ulcers, herpes, allergic rash, hives, shingles, and burns. It is also found in massage balm. The primary external use of snake grass, though, is to treat poisonous insect stings and snake bites.

· · · · ·

SNAKE JASMINE [GOLDEN GRASS]

Rhinacanthus nasutus

tong-pan-châng | thong phan chang

ทองพันชั่ง

TASTE: *Toxic*
PART USED: *Whole plant*

Internal Application: Snake jasmine is used to treat fevers, sore throat, colds, and lung diseases, such as bronchitis and tuberculosis. It lowers blood pressure, and is therefore an effective treatment for hypertension. Tea made from this herb has a laxative effect, helps with back pain, and is useful to encourage passing of gallstones. The Wat Pho texts recommend the leaf as a diuretic, laxative, and anthelmintic (i.e., expels parasites), and as a detoxifying remedy for fever, blood poisoning, skin disease, and cancer. It is said that snake jasmine must be collected between sunset and sunrise because sunlight destroys the potency of the plant.

External Application: A tincture or macerate made of snake jasmine leaves is used topically as a treatment for bacterial and fungal skin infections, rashes, ringworm, and other skin parasites.

· · · · ·

SOAP NUT [SOAP BERRY]

Sapindus rarak

má-kam-dee-kwaai | makhamdikhwai

มะคำดีควาย

TASTE: *Bitter*
PART USED: *Seed, fruit*

Internal Application: The seed of the soap nut tree is traditionally used for treatment of fever and food poisoning, and is considered to be a bitter tonic. The Wat Pho texts mention the pulp of the soap nut fruit as an ingredient in drops to counter ear infection.

External Application: The soap nut fruit was at one time used in South Asia as a natural soap, and still is an ingredient in many natural herbal soaps and shampoos. In Thailand, the soap nut is used medicinally to counter itching of the skin, such as in the case of allergic reactions, hives, rashes, and dandruff. It is also used as a skin tonic and as a remedy for ringworm.

In the West, soap nut can be purchased online, where it is being marketed as a laundry additive.

. . . . .

STAR ANISE
Illicium verum
jan bpàet glèep | chan paet klip
จันทน์แปดกลีบ

TASTE: *Aromatic Pungent*
PART USED: *Seed*

Internal Application: Star anise is mainly a digestive used to counter flatulence, indigestion, irritable bowel, gastritis, and other stomach or intestinal cramping. It is gentle enough to use safely with children and infants. Star anise is a useful cold remedy for cases of dry cough, congestion, flu, and sore throat. As an expectorant, it is especially useful in cases of bronchitis, asthma, and other respiratory infections. It is an excellent remedy for insomnia, and promotes regular menstruation.

External Application: Star anise is beneficial for the heart-mind and is used in oils to calm the Subtle Winds.

Star anise is often used to flavor Thai tea (iced or hot). Just add 2–3 stars to your tea before brewing.

. . . . .

STONEBREAKER
Pyllanthus niruri
lûuk-dtâi-bai | luk tai bai
ลูกใต้ใบ

TASTE: *Bitter*
PART USED: *Whole plant*

Internal Application: Stonebreaker is one of the most useful Bitter plants in the Thai pharmacopeia. It is very beneficial for the kidneys and liver, and is held to be an excellent daily tonic for diabetes and hypoglycemia. It has a calming effect on the circulatory system, lowers blood pressure, and relieves stress, nervousness, insomnia, and anxiety. As a bitter tonic, stonebreaker is prescribed for any type of liver disease, such as hepatitis, cirrhosis, and for cases of jaundice. As an effective diuretic, it is used to treat inflamed kidneys, gall stones, prostate disease, gout, diseases of the pancreas, gonorrhea, venereal disease, excessive or frequent menstruation, as well as cases of infrequent or painful urination.

Stonebreaker is also a tonic for the stomach, easing stomach pains and increasing the appetite. It is frequently prescribed in cases of fever and back pain, and has been shown to be of use as a daily tonic for blood detoxification in cases of AIDS and other blood diseases. The Wat Pho texts also mention stonebreaker as a remedy for vomiting in infants, malaria, and flatulence.

External Application: Stonebreaker may also be used topically to as an antibacterial and vulnerary for wounds, sores, inflammations, or skin infections.

. . . . .

SUGAR APPLE [CUSTARD APPLE, SOURSOP]
Annona squamosa
nói nàa | noina
น้อยหน่า

TASTE: *The leaves are Toxic. The seeds are Toxic and Oily.*
PART USED: *Leaves, seeds*

Internal Application: The seeds of the sugar apple treat parasites.

External Application: The leaves and seeds of the sugar apple tree are ground into powder and used to treat head lice.

The fruit of the sugar apple, which is found in abundance in the markets during its season, is one of the sweetest fruits we have ever tasted.

. . . . .

SUGAR CANE
Saccharum officinarum
ôi | oi
อ้อย

TASTE: *Sweet, Bitter*
PART USED: *Stalk*

Internal Application: Sugar cane treats dehydration so effectively that, while drinking pure fresh sugar cane juice is ideal, even just chewing the fibrous stalk is beneficial. Medicinally, sugar cane is mainly an adjuvant. Fresh cane juice is added to remedies to treat fever, sore throat, cough, congestion, bladder infections, urinary tract infections, low energy, low immunity, chronic disease, chronic fatigue, and emaciation. Raw, unrefined sugar is added to herbal teas that treat fever and lymph problems. Rock sugar is added to treatments for fevers, colds, and sore throat. Sugar as medicine rarely involves highly processed white sugar. The juice of a related plant, the black sugar cane (Saccharum sinense), is a diuretic used in remedies for kidney disorders and venereal diseases.

Sugar cane is commonly available from street vendors all over South Asia. In Thailand, iced sugar cane is sold in bite-sized chunks or in bottles of freshly pressed juice. The cane is chewed, and the woody pulp is spat out when the juice has been extracted. Any way it is ingested, there are few things more pleasurable on a hot sticky day than fresh sugar cane.

. . . . .

SULFUR
gam má tăn | kammathan
กำมะถัน

TASTE: *Toxic*

Internal Application: Pure powdered sulfur is primarily used externally; however, there are some cases where it is used internally to treat toxins.

External Application: Sulfur is applied topically to treat fungal infections, acne, ringworm, scabies, and other skin parasites. It is also commonly used in Thailand to treat mange on dogs.

. . . . .

TAMARIND
Tamarindus indica
má kăam | makham
มะขาม

TASTE: *The leaves are Sour and Astringent. The fruit is Sour, Astringent, and slightly Toxic. The bark is Heating.*
PART USED: *Whole plant*

Internal Application: The seeds of the tamarind are used as a purgative to expel tapeworms and other intestinal parasites, and are also recommended as a tonic for health, strength, and vigor. The fresh juice of the tamarind is the Thai equivalent of the West's prune juice and is a favorite remedy for constipation. It also treats fever.

Tamarind is considered to be a blood purifier, and is recommended for pregnancy and postpartum. Tea made from the young leaves and pods of the tamarind is a laxative, and is also used to treat colds and fevers. The flowers are reputed to lower blood pressure, and the bark is an astringent for diarrhea and fever.

External Application: Used in hot herbal compresses, tamarind leaves expel excess fluid and constrict the tissue. A poultice from the fruit is used externally to reduce fever. The leaves of the tamarind are also frequently used topically to treat skin ulcers and sores. The juice and decoction of the bark are both useful astringents for general antiseptic treatment of the skin, and are frequently applied directly to oily or infected skin before sauna or steam bath. The bark treats inflamed gums, cavities, and some skin parasites.

Tamarind is a common ingredient in Thai cuisine. The pulp of the fruit (available at Thai, Indian, and some Latino groceries) is cooked and added to soups and curries for flavor. The flowers, fruit, and young leaves are eaten in soups and curries. Unripe fruit is also candied with sugar, salt, and red chili flakes and sold by street vendors.

· · · · ·

TI PLANT
Cordyline fruticosa
màak pûu màak mia | makphumakmia
หมากผู้หมากเมีย

TASTE: *Tasteless, Oily, Cooling*
PART USED: *Leaves*

Internal Application: The ti plant primarily treats fever and toxins, but it also is an astringent with a wide range of applications. It is a hemostatic, meaning that it is used traditionally to stop bleeding in cases of bloody vomit, stool, or urine. It is also employed to stop the coughing up of blood associated with tuberculosis, to halt excessive menstruation, and to curtail internal bleeding of the organs, bruises, contusions, and hematoma. The ti plant is also used for treatment of diarrhea, dysentery, arthritis, fever, and measles.

External Application: Topically treats skin irritation from heat and toxicity, and stops bleeding. As a gargle, it is effective against tooth and gum disease, bleeding gums, and halitosis (i.e., bad breath).

· · · · ·

TURMERIC
Curcuma longa
kà-mîn | khamin
ขมิ้น

TASTE: *Astringent, Bitter*
PART USED: *Rhizome*

Internal Application: Turmeric treats diarrhea caused by excess Water Element, moves Wind, and dries mucus. It soothes inflammation and cleans the blood. Turmeric is used as a stimulant for the digestion, and aids in treatment of flatulence, peptic ulcers, indigestion, irritable bowel, and gastritis. For these reasons, it is often used as an adjuvant in preparations for gastrointestinal complaints. It is said to lower blood sugar and is therefore also used for diabetes and hypoglycemia. Turmeric is also a remedy for cough, arthritis, chronic back pain, and painful or blocked menstruation. Turmeric leaves may be used as an antidote for food poisoning and for treatment of hepatitis, as they have a detoxifying effect on the blood, digestive tract, and liver, and regulate the body's secretion of hormones. Turmeric is currently being researched for its anticarcinogenic properties.

External Application: Topically, turmeric is beneficial for the skin and reduces inflammation, especially in the joints. It is frequently found in hot herbal compress formulas, as well as herbal balms and liniments, as it treats the skin and moves Wind. Turmeric treats ringworm and athlete's foot. When applied to wounds, turmeric speeds healing and prevents infection. The turmeric rhizome relives itching and swelling, and has a slight antiseptic effect. It therefore can be used topically on insect bites, rashes, allergic reactions, hives, and superficial wounds. It is also used as an anti-inflammatory for bruises and sprains.

· · · · ·

WAX-LEAVED CLIMBER
Cryptolepis buchanani
tǎo en òn | thao en-on
เถาเอ็นอ่อน

TASTE: *Sweet, Bitter*
PART USED: *Stem, root, leaves*

Internal Application: Internally used as a remedy for fatigue and for mental invigoration. Wax-leaved climber is frequently used to relieve tendon stiffness, as well as muscular aches and pains. It is said to improve circulation.

External Application: Used in compresses, poultices, and liniments to heal tendons and ligaments, to treat strains and sprains, as well as for contusions and other acute injuries.

· · · · ·

WATER MIMOSA
Neptunia oleracea
pàk grà chàyt | phak krachet
ผักกระเฉด

TASTE: *Tasteless, Cooling*
PART USED: *Stalk, leaves*

Internal Application: Water mimosa reduces fever, treats venereal diseases, and eliminates poisons. It moves phlegm, is a tonic that nourishes the body, and relieves headache caused by toxins. Water mimosa also treats food poisoning and allergy.

· · · · · ·

WHITE CLAY
din-sŏr phong | dinsophong
ดินสอพอง

TASTE: *Cooling*

Internal Application: White clay is used internally for drawing out toxins, purging, and treating addictions.

External Application: Topically, many different varieties of clay are used on the skin to soothe skin rashes, hives, insect bites, and irritations.

· · · · · ·

WILD PEPPER LEAF [WILD BETEL, PIPER CHABA]
Piper sarmentosum
chá pluu | cha phlu
ช้าพลู

TASTE: *Spicy/Hot*
PART USED: *Leaves*

Internal Application: Wild pepper leaf is used traditionally to stimulate digestion, to treat flatulence, indigestion, diarrhea, and dysentery, and to ease bloated stomach, abdominal discomfort, and symptoms of irritable bowel and gastritis. It is also employed as a cold remedy, especially in the case of severe lung congestion. Wild pepper leaf treats asthma and works as an expectorant. It also relieves flu, reduces fever, and aids digestion, as well as treating toothache.

External Application: Wild pepper leaf topically treats dermatitis. The wild pepper leaf is well known as a muscle relaxant, and is frequently applied to aches, pains, and sore muscles.

· · · · · ·

WOOLLY GRASS [BLADY GRASS, COGON GRASS]
Imperata cylindrica
yâa-kaa | ya kha
หญ้าคา

TASTE: *Sweet*
PART USED: *Root*

Internal Application: Woolly grass is used primarily as a hemostatic (i.e., to stop bleeding) in cases of blood in the vomit, urine, or phlegm. Its diuretic properties also make it useful in the treatment of fevers, urinary tract infections, kidney disease and stones, bladder problems, cystitis, blood in the urine, vaginal discharge, sexually transmitted diseases, and other urogenital problems.

External Application: Woolly grass is used topically to treat dermatological conditions, including acne and skin infections. It also cleanses and assists with bone setting.

. . . . .

YANAANG
Tilacora triandra
yâa naang | yanang
ย่านาง

TASTE: *Tasteless, Bitter*
PART USED: *Roots, leaves*

Internal Application: This herb is used in the Thai tradition to treat fevers. It is used by some Hill Tribes to treat sprains, bruises, sore muscles, and postpartum to lessen pain and promote healing. Yanaang is extremely effective at counteracting poison.

External Application: Yanaang reduces heat and inflammation and draws out poison. It is found in balms and liniments that promote cooling and that soothe insect bites, prickly heat, and stings. It is beneficial for skin infections, including staphylococcus.

In the West, Yanaang leaves can be readily found in the frozen aisle at Asian food markets.

. . . . .

YLANG YLANG
Canaga odorata
grà-dang-ngaa | kradangnga
กระดังงา

TASTE: *Fragrant/Cool*
PART USED: *Flower*

Internal Application: Ylang ylang flower is a tonic for the heart, and is used traditionally to treat dizziness and fainting spells. It is also a tonic for the blood, and balances the Elements. The leaf and wood are diuretic.

External Application: Added to topical oils or inhalations, ylang ylang calms the Subtle Winds and soothes the heart-mind.

. . . . .

ZEDOARY
Curcumin zedoaria
kà-mîn ôi | khamin-oi
ขมิ้นอ้อย

TASTE: *Spicy/Hot, Astringent*
PART USED: *Rhizome*

Internal Application: Zedoary is beneficial for tendons, tissues, and muscles. Related to turmeric, zedoary is used for similar purposes. It is effective against nausea, vomiting, intestinal cramps, irritable bowel, gastritis, and diarrhea, and is often added as an adjuvant to laxative herbs due to its soothing effect on the stomach. It is also effective against fever, and is used by some Hill Tribes to treat dysentery.

External Application: Topically, zedoary is used in liniments that treat acute injury, especially of tendons, tissue, and muscles. Zedoary is also a topical antiseptic, and is used in the Thai tradition and by some Hill Tribes to treat cuts, wounds, and insect bites.

. . . . .

ZERUMBET GINGER
Zingiber zerumbet
gà-teu | kathue
กะทือ

TASTE: *Bitter*
PART USED: *Rhizome*

Internal Application: Zerumbet ginger has many of the same properties as common ginger, but to a lesser degree. It is used traditionally to treat stomach pain and cramping, as well as food poisoning, allergy, nausea, and vomiting. It can be used successfully to treat irritable bowel, gastritis, and indigestion.

External Application: A tincture of Zerumbet ginger is applied topically to soothe arthritis pains. It is said to give especially good results when massaged into the skin.

Appendices

Wetchasueksa Phaetsatsangkhep
Translated by Tracy Wells

Translator's Introduction

The following is a partial translation of the first volume of a Thai medical text called *The Study of Medicine, Summary of Medical Science* (*Wetchasueksa phaetsatsangkhep* เวชศึกษา แพทย์ศาสตร์สังเขป), a three-volume set published by the School of Traditional Medicine at Wat Phra Chetuphon (commonly known as "Wat Pho" or "Wat Po"). Compiled in the mid-19th century, and first published in 1909, it is a summary of the main texts that form the theoretical foundation of Thai Traditional Medicine (TTM). This text was originally used as a teaching aid in schools where TTM was being taught alongside Western medicine. It is still being used in traditional medical schools in Thailand today. As TTM becomes more well known outside Thailand, there is increasing interest in the history, theory, and practice of this healing art. It is important that the main texts related to the practice of TTM be translated and used as the foundation for understanding TTM theory, since they are an integral part of the tradition.

Stating that skillful medical practitioners must have knowledge of four primary matters, this particular text is divided into four main sections: Pathogenesis of Disease, Identification of Disease, Pharmacology, and Administration of Treatment. Each of these sections offers an opportunity to become familiar with the vocabulary and basic concepts of TTM. Although some sections contain detailed descriptions, often, the text reads more like an outline. This is due to the fact that, traditionally, this material would have been handed down orally. Therefore, a text such as this was probably originally intended to serve as a memory device that would aid students in recalling key concepts encountered while studying directly with a practitioner. This sort of direct experience is the only way to develop a thorough understanding of the concepts presented in the text and to begin to appreciate their practical applications.

As for this translation, my main goal was to stay as true as possible to the source material. The integrity of the original text's outline structure is for the most part maintained. All of the main sections are numbered according to the system used in the original. However, some subheadings and lists contained within the body of the text that do not have numerical designations in the original are numbered here for the sake of clarity. Additionally, some of the longer lists were converted to table form for the same reason. I have also added footnotes for explanatory purposes that do not appear in the original. I have occasionally added information that is missing from the charts or tables in Volume 1 of the source text, when such information can be found in other volumes; those instances have been noted. The inclusion of any other material that does not appear in the original text is indicated by the use of editor's brackets.

There are several challenges inherent in any translation such as this, the largest being to find the right balance between translating word for word (where the inherent meaning often gets lost) and translating for meaning (where the original wording may be sacrificed). I mostly opted for the latter, although I did try to keep as much of the original wording as possible—especially for vocabulary specific to TTM. The first time certain specialized terms appear, I included a translation in all of the pertinent languages—English, romanized Thai, Thai, and, occasionally, Pāli. In these instances, the Thai script was romanized following the Royal Thai General System of Transcription and the Pāli terms were spelled in accordance with the spelling given in the Pāli Text Society dictionary. Thereafter, these terms are referred to only in English, capitalized in order to indicate that it is traditional medical terminology.

There were several additional complexities encountered in this translation, mostly having to do with the names for various diseases and plants. As much as possible, I tried to avoid using modern medical interpretations of the various diseases mentioned in the text, instead choosing to define medical terms by the meanings that traditional practitioners most likely used at the time this text was compiled. With regards to the various medicinal components mentioned in the text, scientific and English common names are given when available. However, these names may be misleading, since often there may be one plant with several names, or several different plants may all have the same name. This is probably due to the names of plants mentioned in the text being transferred to other plants with similar properties at some point when the original plants became more difficult to find or became extinct. I used several references, including Thai dictionaries, government publications, and university databases, to try to ascertain the most appropriate names for the plants referred to in this text. I also consulted with Wit Sukhsamran, a practitioner of TTM, and relied extensively upon his experience with the the plants and how they are used medicinally.

What has been omitted from this translation should also be mentioned here. I chose to omit many of the remarks concerned with Thai language usage throughout the piece as this translation is chiefly aimed at non-Thai speakers. Since a large portion of the original Preface deals with various issues of semantics, I have cut most of it; however, I did retain a translation of the four main category headings, because they offer a succinct overview of the content found in the rest of the text. A list of 82 formulas for medicine and a set of ethical guidelines for medical practitioners have also been left out of this translation. Aside from these omissions, which have been marked with [...] in the translation that follows, all of the content contained in the major sections of the main body of the original text is included below.

Late in the production of this translation, I became aware of a 1979 article on TTM by Jean Mulholland that contains material similar to that found in the *Wetchasueksa* text. I did not consult that article in the preparation of this particular translation for two reasons. First, the information cited in the article draws from several different TTM manuals, including a set of guidelines for examination in TTM theory and pharmacy, as well as several classical textbooks of traditional medicine and pharmacy. While that material bears a resemblance to the material found in the *Wetchasueksa* text, its presentation in the article does not strictly follow the outline structure of this particular text. Second, while most of the main sections included in the *Wetchasueksa* text are mentioned in the article, there are several subsections that are omitted. The translation I have prepared, on the other hand, specifically aims to reflect the format and content of the original *Wetchasueksa* text by keeping the structure of the source material as intact as possible.

It is my deepest hope that this translation will be of some benefit as a reference for those with an interest in TTM. However, I am not a physician in either the traditional or modern sense of the word, and the material presented here is not intended as a substitute for consulting a trained physician, since all matters regarding health require medical supervision. Also, any mistakes or misinterpretations that may lie herein are completely my own and should not in any way reflect upon my teachers, the teachings, or the tradition from which they come.

I would like to thank all of my Thai language teachers, especially the teachers at University of Wisconsin-Madison Southeast Asian Studies Summer Institute (SEASSI), as well as Narisa Naropakorn. I am also thankful for my Thai massage teachers—both near and far—for nurturing my initial interest in the traditional healing arts of Thailand. And special thanks go to Wit Sukhsamran, who spent countless hours patiently going over minute details of this text with me. Despite a busy schedule, he was always willing to answer questions or shed light on particularly challenging passages. His many contributions are not individually cited throughout the translation. Instead, I will just hope it suffices to say that this translation would not have been possible without his help.

Most importantly, credit for this translation must be given to Thailand, Thai tradition, and the Thai people, whose recognition of the importance of texts such as this has ensured that the wisdom of this traditional knowledge is imparted to each new generation of TTM practitioners.

The Study of Medicine, Summary of Medical Science

Preface

[...]

Medical practitioners who will be skillful in treating disease must know about four primary matters:

1. Pathogenesis of Disease [literally, "origin of disease"]
2. Identification of Disease
3. Pharmacology [literally, "medicinal substances for treating disease"]
4. Administration of Treatment [literally, "appropriate medicine for correctly treating a specific disease"]

1. Pathogenesis of Disease

The Pathogenesis of Disease is divided into four aspects:

1. Elemental Causative Factor (*that samutthan* ธาตุสมุฏฐาน)
2. Seasonal Causative Factor (*utu samutthan* อุตุสมุฏฐาน)
3. Age Causative Factor (*ayu samutthan* อายุสมุฏฐาน)
4. Time Causative Factor (*kanla samutthan* กาลสมุฏฐาน)

1.1. Elemental Causative Factor

The Elemental Causative Factor refers to the place where the Elements become established, with the Elements being divided into four groups:

1. Earth [Element] Causative Factor (*pathawi samutthan* ปถวีสมุฏฐาน)
2. Water [Element] Causative Factor (*apo samutthan* อาโปสมุฏฐาน)
3. Wind [Element] Causative Factor (*wayo samutthan* วาโยสมุฏฐาน)
4. Fire [Element] Causative Factor (*techo samutthan* เตโชสมุฏฐาน)

Altogether, there are 42 Elemental Causative Factors, or as they are also called, the Four Elements of Earth, Water, Wind and Fire, which are further explained below.

Earth Element (*pathawi that* ปถวีธาตุ), Twenty Types
1. Hair of the Head
2. Hair of the Body—i.e., eyebrows, mustache, beard
3. Nails—fingernails and toenails
4. Teeth—incisors, canines, and molars—20 primary teeth, 32 permanent teeth
5. Skin—According to the texts, it is understood to mean the exterior covering of the body that has three layers: thick skin, middle skin, and outer skin. But, in reality, skin such as that in the mouth is one more type of skin called wet skin.
6. Muscle—layers of round muscle tissue and flat muscle tissue throughout the body
7. Tendons, Ligaments, Blood Vessels, and Nerves[1]
8. Bone—cartilage and bone
9. Bone Marrow
10. Kidney
11. Heart
12. Liver—[meaning] liver and pancreas
13. Membrane [i.e., fascia][2]— connective tissue throughout the body that has the ability to be elastic and flexible
14. Spleen
15. Lungs[3]
16. Large Intestine
17. Small Intestine
18. Undigested Food[4]—undigested food in stomach
19. Waste—waste coming from the small intestines, in the lower intestines, excreted through the anus
20. Brain and Spinal Nervous Tissue

[...]

Water Element (*apothat* อาโปธาตุ), Twelve Types
1. Bile (*pittang* ปิตตํ), divided into two kinds: – Bound Bile (*phattha pitta* พัทธปิตตํ)—bile in the gallbladder – Unbound Bile (*aphattha pitta* อพัทธปิตตํ)—bile outside the gallbladder that flows into the small intestines
2. Mucus (*semhang* เสมํหํ), divided three ways: – Mucus in the Neck and Head (*so semha* สอเสมหะ) – Mucus in the Chest (*ura semha* อุรเสมหะ) – Mucus that is Below the Navel to the Anus (*khut semha* คูธเสมหะ)[5]
3. Pus
4. Blood (*lohitang* โลหิตํ)[6]—arterial blood and venous blood
5. Sweat
6. Fat
7. Tears
8. Oil—oil, sebum, or lymph
9. Saliva
10. Nasal Mucus—clear fluid in nose and throat
11. Synovial Fluid—joint lubricant
12. Urine

Wind Element (*wayothat* วาโยธาตุ), Six Types
1. Wind that Moves from the Feet to the Head, or from the stomach to the throat, as in belching, etc.
2. Wind that Moves from the Head to the Feet, or from the small intestines to the anus, as in flatulence, etc.
3. Wind that Moves in the Abdomen, outside the digestive tract
4. Wind that Moves in the Intestines and Stomach
5. Wind that Moves Throughout the Entire Body (*lom* ลม)[7]
6. Wind that is Inhaled and Exhaled—breath

Fire Element (*techothat* เตโชธาตุ), Four Types
1. Fire that Warms the Body, maintaining regular body temperature
2. Fire that Makes a Feeling of Heat, creating a sense of unrest that makes it necessary to bathe and be fanned[8]
3. Fire that Causes Aging and Decay
4. Fire that Digests Food

The names of the Twenty Earth Elements, Twelve Water Elements, Six Wind Elements, and Four Fire Elements that have been outlined [above] are the places where disease becomes established. This occurs when the Four Elements (*that tang si* ธาตุทั้ง ๔) become altered or deviate from a natural state (*wikan* วิกาล). This is explained in the classical texts *Khamphi that wiphang* (คัมภีร์ธาตุวิภังค์) and *Khamphi roknithan* (คัมภีร์โรคนิทาน).

Medical practitioners know the place where disease becomes established according to the condition or symptoms (*akan* อาการ) of the Four Elements, as well as the Medicinal components (*tua ya* ตัวยา) that cure disease, as categorized in the text *Khamphi roknithan*. Here, only the names of the Four Elements are given, since this is just a summary.

When the 42 Elements become altered or deviate from a natural state, they are divided into three groups of Elemental Causative Factors:

1. **Bile** (Th. *pitta* ปิตตะ; Pāli *pitta*)[9] Disease-causing Factor: Sickness due to Bile
2. **Mucus** (Th. *semha* เสมหะ; Pāli *semha*) Disease-causing Factor: Sickness due to Mucus
3. **Wind** (Th. *wata* วาต; Pāli *vāta*) Disease-causing Factor: Sickness due to Wind

When all three groups of Causative Factors come together, it is called Combined Disease (*sannibatika aphatha* สันนิบาติกาอาพาธา)—that is, sickness due to the offenses (*thot* โทษ) coming together (*sannibat* สันนิบาต).

These three groups of Causative Factors frequently become altered or deviate from a natural state. When there are abnormal seasonal variations, the three groups of Causative Factors become altered at that time. This will be explained further next.

1.2. Seasonal Causative Factor

Sickness can arise when the seasons change; therefore, the seasons are a cause of disease. The classical medical texts divide the seasons in three ways: "Three Seasons," "Four Seasons," or "Six Seasons."

Three Seasons

Hot Season (*khim ha ruedu* คิมหะฤดู or *khim hanta ruedu* คิมหันตฤดู)	1st day of waning moon of 4th month, to 1st day of waning moon of 8th month[10]	– Causes heat – Rainy and cold weather mix – Fire Element is the Causative Factor, [specifically][11] Fire that Warms the Body
Rainy Season (*wasanta ruedu* วสันตฤดู)[12]	1st day of waning moon of 8th month, to 1st day of waning moon of 12th month	– Causes coolness – Cold and hot weather mix – Wind Element is the Causative Factor, [specifically] Wind that Moves in the Abdomen, outside the digestive tract
Cold Season (*hemanta ruedu* เหมันตฤดู)	1st day of waning moon of 12th month, to 1st day of waning moon of 4th month	– Causes coldness – Hot and rainy weather mix – Water Element is the Causative Factor, specifically Mucus, Blood

With the change of seasons, there are variations of hot and cold weather mixing together. This [fluctuation] causes humans to become ill—due to the relationship of the outer Elements and the bodily Elements being unequal. When one season follows the other, the seasonal variation causes the internal bodily Elements to become irregular. When the circulation of [bodily] Elements does not keep pace with the season, then illness will occur.

Four Seasons

One year is divided into four seasons. Each season is three months.

First Season	1st day of waning moon of 4th month, to full moon of 7th month	Fire Element is the Causative Factor
Second Season	1st day of waning of moon 7th month, to full moon of 10th month	Wind Element is the Causative Factor
Third Season	1st day of waning moon of 10th month, to full moon of 1st month	Water Element is the Causative Factor
Fourth Season	1st day of waning moon of 1st month, to full moon of 4th month	Earth Element is the Causative Factor

Six Seasons

One year is divided into six seasons. Each season is two months.

First Season	1st day of waning moon of 4th month, to full moon of 6th month	Illness caused by Fire Element, [specifically] Bile, Body Heat (*kamdao* กำเดา)
Second Season	1st day of waning moon of 6th month, to full moon of 8th month	Illness caused by combination of Fire Element, Wind Element, Body Heat
Third Season	1st day of waning moon of 8th month, to full moon of 10th month	Illness caused by Wind Element and Mucus
Fourth Season	1st day of waning moon of 10th month, to full moon of 12th month	Illness caused by Wind, Mucus, Urine
Fifth Season	1st day of waning moon of 12th month, to full moon of 2nd month	Illness caused by Mucus, Body Heat, Blood
Sixth Season	1st day of waning moon of 2nd month, to full month of 4th month	Illness caused by Earth Element, Combination of Blood, Wind, Body Heat, Mucus

1.3. Age Causative Factor

Age Causative Factor is divided into three phases.

Phase	Age	Causative Factor
1. Early Age (*pathommawai* ปฐมวัย)	Birth–16 yrs.	Water Element—specifically Mucus, Blood
	– Birth–8 yrs.	Mucus is the Dominant Element (*chao ruean* เจ้าเรือน), with aspects of Blood
	– 8–16 yrs.	Blood is the Dominant Element[13], with aspects of Mucus
2. Middle Age (*matchimawai* มัชฌิมวัย)	16–32 yrs.	Water Element—specifically two parts Blood, and one part Wind
3. Old Age (*patchimwai* ปัจฉิมวัย)	32–64 yrs.	Wind Element
	64 yrs. and up	Wind Element is Dominant Element, with aspects of Water, specifically Mucus, Sweat

1.4. Time Causative Factor

Time Causative Factor is divided into four periods during the day and four periods during the night.[14]

First Period	dawn–9 AM	Water Element is the Causative Factor, specifically Mucus
	dusk–9 PM	
Second Period[15]	9 AM–noon	Water Element is the Causative Factor, specifically Blood
	9 PM–midnight	
Third Period	noon–3 PM	Water Element is the Causative Factor, specifically Bile
	midnight–3 AM	
Fourth Period	3 PM–dusk	Wind Element is the Causative Factor
	3 AM–dawn	

1.5. Geographic Causative Factor

Following what has already been said—that is, the four Causative Factors that contribute to disease as listed above—according to the classical medical text *Khamphi samutthan winitchai* (คัมภีร์สมุฏฐานวินิจฉัย), one additional Disease-causing Factor is the region where one is born or where one resides. Therefore, region or habitat is categorized here as a Geographic Causative Factor (*prathet samutthan* ประเทศสมุฏฐาน).

Wherever one resides, the Elements that are established within the body become accustomed to the environment or atmosphere of that region. Changing habitats or environments—for example, moving from highlands to lowlands or from hot climates to cold climates—can cause one to fall ill if not acclimated to the new environment. People who move from the seaside to the highland forest, or vice-versa, may get sick, which really is just due to the unfamiliar water or unfamiliar atmosphere. It is really nothing but the Elements being unfamiliar, even if the person has lived in the new environment for a long time. The mud can occasionally be polluted, which is why this particular disease arises. Medical practitioners of all sorts will therefore recommend going to an unpolluted place to recover. Due to these reasons, region or habitat is categorized as a Causative Factor that contributes to the occurrence of disease.

Geographic Causative Factor, Four Types

Birthplace	Region	Causative Factor
1. Highland, upland	Hot Region (*prathet ron* ประเทศร้อน)	Fire Element
2. Rocky, desert-like terrain	Warm Region (*prathet un* ประเทศอุ่น)	Water Element, [specifically] Bile, Blood
3. Wetland	Cool Region (*prathet yen* ประเทศเย็น)	Wind Element
4. Saltwater wetland	Cold Region (*prathet nao* ประเทศหนาว)	Earth Element

Characteristics of Symptoms

The diseases that occur in humans arise in the 32 Parts of the Body (*akan samsipsong* อาการ ๓๒)[16] —that is, the Hair of the Head, Hair of the Body, and so on. When a disease occurs in any part of the body, it is called by that part of the body followed by the word Distortion (*phikan* พิการ). This describes the Causative Factor, referring to the origin of the disease. When any one of the bodily Elements of Water, Wind, or Fire becomes irregular, it gives rise to disease.[17] That part of the body is then called Distorted, which indicates the Causative Factor. The examination of the Causative Factors in order to identify the illness and the factor that gives rise to the disease is done by way of investigating the Elemental, Seasonal, Age, Time, and Geographic Causative Factors that have been described above. When a doctor applies a remedy, the remedy must accurately follow those Causative Factors. But, when a doctor examines a patient with certain symptoms, understands that it is a particular disease—i.e., a cold (*wat* หวัด), Wasting Disease (*kasai* กษัย), fever (*khai* ไข้)—and applies a remedy according [just] to the name of the disease, it is not accurately following the characteristics of the Causative Factors. This is because the name is [just] a conventional name that doctors have called the disease throughout the generations. But diseases that are rarely found, or something with similar symptoms, might be called different names by different doctors. If you are going to accurately apply a remedy, you must consider the Causative Factors. In the classical text *Khamphi that wiphang*, the conventional names for diseases are not used; instead, diseases are called by the Causative Factor. For example, when symptoms of disease in the liver are observed, it is called Distortion of the Liver; in the lungs, it is called Distortion of the Lungs; when disease is due to Mucus, it is called Distortion of the Mucus. This allows students of medicine to know the symptoms accurately.

The symptom characteristics describe the main Causative Factor, which is a tool for the doctor who is listening carefully during an examination. The types of diseases that humans most often have are in three groups—that is, disease that occurs due to Bile, disease that occurs due to Mucus, and disease that occurs due to Wind, as has already been explained in the [section on] Elemental Causative Factors.

Distorted Earth Element Causative Factors
(*samutthan pathawi phikan* สมุฏฐานปถวีพิการ)

Distortion of:	Symptoms:
Hair of the Head	Painful scalp; loss of scalp hair
Hair of the Body	Painful skin; loss of body hair [i.e., folliculitis]
Nails	Pain at nail; loss of nails; pus at nails [i.e., nail infection]
Teeth	Severe gum infection; abscessed molar causing pain at the tooth root; cavity
Skin	Itchy skin; rough or brittle skin; burning skin
Muscle	Flesh that is rash-like and burning; flesh that is mole-like or wart-like; [flesh] that is bruised or has dark marks
Tendons, Ligaments, Blood Vessels, and Nerves	Feeling emotionally tied-up, anxious, or faint; [feeling] weak or empty [i.e., bodily discomforts]
Bone	Affliction at the bones [i.e., bone disorders]
Bone Marrow	Thickening of bone marrow; beriberi (*nepcha* เหน็บชา, lit. "numbness and tingling")
Kidney	Hot and cold shivers; Wasting Disease
Heart	Bad mood; touchiness; anger
Liver	Enlarged liver; soft or weakened liver; liver abscess; bruised liver
Membrane	Depletion in the lungs; thirst; drying of tissue in the pleura [i.e., tuberculosis with progressive anemia] (*ritsiduang haeng* ริดสีดวงแห้ง)
Spleen	Physical obstruction in chest; tightness in chest; abdominal distention; fatigue
Lungs	Thirst; sensation of warmth in the chest; serious asthma or gasping for breath; very serious disease of the lungs
Large Intestine	Diarrhea; feeling of tightness or firmness in abdomen; constriction of the intestine
Small Intestine	Burping and yawning; bloody stool; an unfocused or cloudy look; extreme soreness at waist; sharp, shooting bilateral abdominal pain; sensation of heat in the stomach; burning-like sensation from abdomen to throat [i.e., heartburn]; foul-smelling stool with pus
Undigested Food	Diarrhea; abdominal discomfort; nausea; hiccups
Waste	Irregular stool; disturbed digestion; diseases such as hemorrhoids (*ritsiduang* ริดสีดวง)
Brain and Spinal Nervous Tissue	Hearing loss; unfocused or cloudy vision; unclear speech; inability to move

Distorted Water Element Causative Factors
(*samutthan apo phikan* สมุฏฐานอาโปพิการ)

Distortion of:	Symptoms:
1. **Bile** a. Bound Bile b. Unbound Bile	a. Delirium b. Pain in head; internal feeling of heat; hot and cold shakes; yellow eyes; yellow urine; fever
2. **Mucus** a. Mucus in Neck and Head b. Mucus in the Chest c. Mucus below the Navel to the Anus	a. Sore throat; dry throat; asthma b. Physical wasting; abdominal rigidity; burning in throat; depletion in lungs c. Mucus or blood in stool
3. **Pus**	Loss of appetite; emaciation
4. **Blood**	Fever; delirium; incoherent speech; red urine; small inflamed elevations on skin or rashes; birthmarks that are black or red; Toxic Diseases (*kanla rok* กาฬโรค)[18]
5. **Sweat**	Dizziness; internal feeling of coolness; easily upset or depressed
6. **Fat**	Skin rash in a circular shape; burning skin; skin that is hot to the touch; secretions of lymph or yellow sebum
7. **Tears**	Filmy covering over eyes; teary eyes; watery eyes; cataracts
8. **Oil**	Yellow skin; yellow eyes; diarrhea
9. **Saliva**	Sore throat; pimples or bumps on tongue
10. **Nasal Mucus**	Pain in the head; unfocused or cloudy vision; nasal drip
11. **Synovial Fluid**	Joint pain; bone pain
12. **Urine**	Urine that is white, yellow, black, red

Distorted Wind Element Causative Factors
(*samutthan wayo phikan* สมุฏฐานวาโยพิการ)

Distortion of:	Symptoms:
1. Wind that Moves from the Feet to the Head	Tremors in the hands and feet; sensation of heat in the abdomen; agitation; yawning and belching; excess of Mucus
2. Wind that Moves from the Head to the Feet	Inability to lift arms and legs; fatigue or stiffness in the joints
3. Wind that Moves in the Abdomen, outside of intestinal tract	Rumbling or gurgling in the abdomen; faintness or dizziness; fatigue or stiffness in the joints
4. Wind that Moves in the Intestines and Stomach	Discomfort in chest; abdominal discomfort; vomiting; nausea; fermented odor
5. Wind that Moves Throughout the Entire Body	Blurry vision; dizziness; bilateral pain in upper thigh area; pain in spine; dry heaves; inability to eat; fever with chills
6. Wind that is Inhaled and Exhaled	Inability to get a deep breath; short or shallow breathing

Distorted Fire Element Causative Factors
(*samutthan techo phikan* สมุฏฐานเตโชพิการ)

Distortion of:	Symptoms:
1. Fire that Warms the Body	Clamminess
2. Fire that Makes a Feeling of Heat	Stiffness in ankle and wrist joints; sickness in lungs; cough; soreness on palms of hands and soles of feet; abdominal rigidity; nausea
3. Fire that Causes Aging and Decay	Lack of sensation in body; inability of the tongue to perceive taste; hearing loss; forehead tension. These symptoms may be intermittent.
4. Fire that Digests Food	Feeling of heat both internally and externally; cold hands; cold feet; perspiration

[Behaviors that Contribute to the Origin of Disease]

Having already mentioned the five Causative Factors, now the behaviors that contribute to the origin of disease will be mentioned in brief. Humans should behave in such a way that does not violate the body. The following are considered to be violations of the body. Violations occur via:

1. [**Food**]: Food is the most important way to take care of the body. Carelessness with what is consumed [consists of] eating too much, not eating enough, eating spoiled food or food that is supposed to be thoroughly cooked but is not cooked all the way, and eating at an

inappropriate time, i.e., by eating food at breakfast that is normally consumed in the afternoon. The consumption of food in this manner disturbs the Elements in the body. This is called: Disease Arising from Food.

2. **Body Movements or Posture:** There are four body positions that should be alternated between: sitting, lying down, standing, and walking. Any movement or posture done to excess will not use the body's Tendons, Ligaments, Blood Vessels, and Nerves in a way that encourages variety. The Tendons, Ligaments, Blood Vessels, and Nerves will deviate from a normal position, causing disease to arise. This is called: Disease Arising from Body Movements or Posture.

3. **Hot and Cold:** Disease can be caused by going from a hot place to an overly cold place; going from the shade into full sun without protection; going from the open-air to a muggy place; going into the rain and getting thoroughly soaked. This is called: Disease Arising from Hot and Cold.

4. **Being Deprived of Sleep, Food, or Water:** Not sleeping at night; not eating at mealtimes; not drinking when thirsty. Enduring deprivation causes disease. This is called: Disease Arising from Being Deprived of Sleep, Food, or Water.

5. **Suppression of Defecation or Urination:** Restraining bowel movements or urination results in an over-accumulation and fluctuation from what is normal. This abnormality can cause the Elements in the body to fluctuate also, which can cause disease. This is called: Disease Arising from Suppression of Defecation or Urination.

6. **Overexertion:** Overexertion is lifting, carrying, hauling, or dragging things that are too heavy for your level of strength. Running, jumping, or overly vigorous exercise vibrates and moves the organs more than usual and displaces them. Working or thinking in an overly focused way can wear you out and use all of your strength, which can cause disease. This is called Disease Arising from Overexertion.

7. **Extreme Sadness:** People suffering from excessive sadness have forgotten how to find joy in things that used to be pleasurable—the utmost being when food no longer has any flavor. Then the Nutriment (*namliang* น้ำเลี้ยง) in the body that is bright and clear becomes turbid and muddy, ultimately drying up, depleting the body and causing disease. This is called: Disease Arising from Extreme Sadness.

8. **Extreme Anger:** People who are always angry do not have the clarity of mind to control their temper, which takes a toll on the physical body. Lack of self-control is neglectful of the body, is self-defeating, and allows disease to arise. This is called Disease Arising from Extreme Anger.

2. Identification of Disease

Medical practitioners must know the names of diseases.[19] When patients have symptoms of an illness, many practitioners will identify the disease by saying "you have a cold, a cough, a fever, a disease of Wind," and so on. And there are many other names of diseases that are explained in the classical medical texts.

These names of diseases have been given so that practitioners can determine that when patients have symptoms like this, then it is this disease; with symptoms like that, then it is that disease.

However, in the classical text *Khamphi roknithan*, the name of the disease is not just stated as such. Instead, the name of each Element is given and then followed by the word "Distortion" or "Permanent Break (*taek pai* แตกไป)" which causes the various symptoms of illness. Therefore, these diseases exist when the 42 Elements become Distorted or Broken, which is the reason that humans become sick.

If a disease is to be named strictly according to the facts, then the 42 Elements must be in the name of the disease. For example: Distortion of the Hair of the Head Disease, Distortion of the Teeth Disease, Distortion of the Mucus Disease, Distortion of the Blood Disease, and so on. The word "Disease" in this case means the Element that is Distorted.

If a disease is to be named concisely, then there would be just five ways to name the disease, based on the origin of disease in the five sense organs, that is:

1. Diseases of the Eye (*chakkhu ro kho* จักขุโรโค)
2. Diseases of the Ear (*sot ro kho* โสตโรโค)
3. Diseases of the Nose (*khan ro kho* ฆานโรโค)
4. Diseases of the Tongue (*chioha ro kho* ชิวหาโรโค)
5. Diseases of the Body (*kai ro kho* กายโรโค)

Sense Organ Where Disease Occurs	[Examples of Disease]
Diseases of the Eye	Eyes that are red; eyes that are watery; eyes that have chronic sores
Diseases of the Ear	Deafness [literally, "ears that are deaf"]; hearing loss [literally, "ears that are deficient"]; ear abscess
Diseases of the Nose	Nose sores
Diseases of the Tongue	Tongue that is fissured; tongue ulcers
Diseases of the Body – Diseases of the External Body (*phahit tha ro kho* พหิทธโรโค)	Fungal infection of skin [i.e., tinea versicolor or ringworm]; malignant or nonmalignant chronic ulcerated sores [i.e., cancerous or noncancerous growths]; tropical infection of the skin [i.e., yaws]; leprosy; ulcerated sores

Sense Organ Where Disease Occurs	[Examples of Disease]
Diseases of the Body – Diseases of the Internal Body (*anta ro kho* อันตโรโค)	Fever; [diseases of] Wind; abdominal rigidity; localized abdominal rigidity; abdominal discomfort; stomach discomfort; dysentery; severe diarrhea; tuberculosis

Diseases cannot just be called by a single name since there are names that are given that may vary according to the village or the region. For example, a disease may have the same symptoms, but Northerners may have one name for it, Southerners may have another name, and the classical text may have a different name—even though it is the very same disease. It is not the names of the diseases that need to be amended, rather it is the responsibility of the practitioner to listen carefully and adapt when healing disease within that particular population.

It is recommended for students who are studying to be a doctor to specifically know the various characteristics and symptoms of Toxic Fevers (*khai takkasila* ไข้ตักศิลา). These are known as Toxic Diseases, and they are explained in the classical text *Khamphi takkasila* (คัมภีร์ตักศิลา) that was published in the [text] *Phaetsat songkhro* (แพทย์ศาสตร์สงเคราะห์). Doctors should consider these important fevers.

3. Pharmacology

Doctors must know everything about what is compounded into medicine for treating disease. In order to know the medicines, there are four aspects:

1. Individual Medicinal Components (*tua ya* ตัวยา)
2. Properties of Medicine (*sapphakhun ya* สรรพคุณยา)
3. Multiple Medicinal Ingredients (*khrueang ya* เครื่องยา)—mixed together [acting as a single substance] and called by one name (*phikat ya* พิกัดยา)
4. Methods for Compounding Medicine (*kan prung ya* การปรุงยา)

3.1. Individual Medicinal Components

3.1.1. Identifying Individual Medicinal Components

In order to know the Individual Medicinal Components, it is required to know five things:

– Form
– Color
– Aroma[20]
– Taste
– Name

3.1.2. Raw Materials for Medicine

There are three sorts of raw materials for medicine:

1. Vegetative material (*phuet watthu* พืชวัตถุ): plants, grasses, vines
2. Animal material (*sat watthu* สัตว์วัตถุ): animal body parts
3. Mineral material (*that watthu* ธาตุวัตถุ): various minerals

1. Plants
Plants—Flowers, Pollen or stamen, Fruit, Seeds, Sapwood or inside of bark, Resin, Heartwood, Root. Grasses, Vines

2. Animal Body Parts
Hair or fur, Skin, Antler or horn, Horn[21], Tusk, Fang, Tooth, Molar, Hoof, Bone, Bile

3. Minerals [22]
Camphor (*karabun* การบูร, *Cinnamomum camphora*), Potassium nitrate, Sulfur, Copper sulfate

In order to know the form, color, aroma, and taste of a medicinal substance, you must be able to look at a sample of the real thing at a school, a garden, or other places that have fresh samples. You must study the real thing—both dried and fresh—and become experienced with it. Furthermore, plants from one region might be called one way, and then you might come across a different region calling it another way. Students must investigate in this way in order to become more experienced and knowledgeable.

3.2. Properties of Medicine

3.2.1. Three Medicinal Tastes (*rot ya* รสยา)

There are Three Medicinal Tastes:

1. Medicine with the Cool Taste Property (*ya rot yen* ยารสเย็น)
2. Medicine with the Hot Taste Property (*ya rot ron* ยารสร้อน)
3. Medicine with the Mild Taste Property (*ya rot sukhum* ยารสสุขุม)

1. Medicine with the Cool Taste Property[23]
Medicine made from—Leaves (that are not hot), Pollen, stamen, and pistil, "Seven Antlers or Horns," "Nine Teeth," Ash reduction
Examples: Great Dark Blue Medicine (*ya mahanin* ยามหานิล), Great Black Medicine (*ya mahakan* ยามหากาฬ)
For curing Fire

2. Medicine with the Hot Taste Property
Medicine made from—"Five Families," "Three Pungents," Hatsakhun หัศคุณ (*Micromelum minutum*), Ginger (*khing* ขิง, *Zingiber officinale*), Galangal (*kha* ข่า, *Alpinia galanga, syn. Languas galanga*)
Examples: All [of the medicine called] Yellow Medicine (*ya lueang* ยาเหลือง)
For curing Wind

3. Medicine with the Mild Taste Property
Medicine made from—Kot (โกฐ)[24], Thian (เทียน)[25], Eaglewood or agarwood (*kritsana* กฤษณา, *Aquilaria crassna* or *Aquilaria malaccensis*), Kalamphak กะลำพัก (*Euphorbia antiquorum*), Chalut ชะลูด (*Alyxia reinwardtii*), Cinnamon (*opchoei* อบเชย, *Cinnamomum sp.*), Khondok ขอนดอก (*Asclepias gigantea*), Sandalwood (*chan thet* จันทน์เทศ, *Santalum album*)[26]
Examples: All of the [medicine called] Fragrant Medicine (*ya hom* ยาหอม)
For curing Blood

3.2.2. Nine Medicinal Tastes
Another way to classify the Medicinal Tastes is according to the Nine Medicinal Tastes:

1. Astringent Taste (*rot fat* รสฝาด)	Binds
2. Sweet Taste (*rot wan* รสหวาน)	Permeates the tissue
3. Toxic Taste (*rot mao buea* รสเมาเบื่อ)	Remedies Poison (*phit* พิษ)[27]
4. Bitter Taste (*rot khom* รสขม)	Remedies Blood
5. Spicy-Hot Taste (*rot phet ron* รสเผ็ดร้อน)	Remedies Wind
6. Oily Taste (*rot man* รสมัน)	Remedies Tendons, Ligaments, Blood Vessels, and Nerves
7. Fragrant-Cool Taste (*rot hom yen* รสหอมเย็น)	Refreshes
8. Salty Taste (*rot khem* รสเค็ม)	Permeates the skin
9. Sour Taste (*rot priao* รสเปรี้ยว)	Cuts Mucus
— Tasteless (*rot chuet* รสจืด)	Remedies Mucus

3.2.3. Medicinal Tastes for Elemental Distortions

One more way of classifying [the Medicinal Tastes] is organized according to the Four Elements—i.e., when an Element is Distorted, which Medicinal Taste cures the disease:

Disease arising from:	Responds to:
1. Distorted Earth Element	Astringent Taste Bitter Taste Sweet Taste Oily Taste
2. Distorted Water Element	Bitter Taste Sour Taste Toxic Taste
3. Distorted Fire Element	Tasteless Cool Taste
4. Distorted Wind Element	Mild Taste Spicy-Hot Taste

Teaching these Properties of Medicine in a complete and detailed way is a difficult activity. Therefore, in order to obtain more extensive knowledge, students must study the large texts, such as the text about Properties of Medicine, *Khamphi sapphakhun* (คัมภีร์สรรพคุณ).

3.3. Multiple Medicinal Ingredients

[These are] mixed together [acting as a single substance] and called by one name. Categorized into groups by rank (*phikat* พิกัด). Examples to follow.[28]

Two Entities Group

Name	Individual Medicinal Components	Part Used
Two Perfumes (*thawekhantha* ทเวคันธา)	Ironwood (*bunnak* บุนนาค, *Mesua ferrea* GUTTIFERAE)	Root
	Masang มะทราง (*Madhuca pierrei* SAPOTACEAE)	Root
Two Perfumes of Three Things (*thawetrikhantha* ทเวตรีคันธา)	Ironwood (*bunnak* บุนนาค, *Mesua ferrea* GUTTIFERAE)	Flower, Heart-wood, Root
	Masang มะทราง (*Madhuca pierrei* SAPOTACEAE)	Flower, Heart-wood, Root

Three Entities Group

Name	Individual Medicinal Components	Part Used
Three Medicines that are Very Fragrant (*trisukhon* ตรีสุคนธ์)[29]	Cinnamon (*opchoei thet* อบเชยเทศ, *Cinnamomum verum*, syn. *Cinnamomum zeylanicum* LAURACEAE)	Root
	"Thai cinnamon" (*opchoei thai* อบเชยไทย, *Cinnamomum bejolghota* or *Cinnamomum iners* LAURACEAE)	Root
	Patchouli (*phimsen ton* พิมเสนต้น, *Pogostemon cablin* LABIATAE)	Root
Three Fruits (*triphala* ตรีผลา)	Haritaki (*samo apphaya* สมออัพพยา, *Terminalia chebula* COMBRETACEAE)[30]	Fruit
	Bibhitaki (*samo phiphek* สมอพิเภก, *Terminalia bellerica* COMBRETACEAE)	Fruit
	Amalaki (*makham pom* มะขามป้อม, *Phyllanthus emblica* PHYLLANTHACEAE)	Fruit
Three Pungents (*trikatuk* ตรีกฏุก)	Black pepper (*phrik thai* พริกไทย, *Piper nigrum* PIPERACEAE)	Seed
	Long pepper (*di pli* ดีปลี, *Piper longum* PIPERACEAE)	Fruit[31]
	Ginger (*khing* ขิง, *Zingiber officinale* ZINGIBERACEAE)	Rhizome
Three Strong Medicines (*trisan* ตรีสาร)[32]	Wild pepper (*cha phlu* ช้าพลู, *Piper sarmentosum* PIPERACEAE)	Root
	Plumbago (*chetta mun phloeng* เจตมูลเพลิง, *Plumbago* sp. PLUMBAGINACEAE)	Root
	Sakhan สะค้าน (*Piper interruptum* PIPERACEAE)	Vine
Three Celestial Waters (*trithanthip* ตรีธารทิพย์)	Banyan tree (*sai yoi* ไทรย้อย, *Ficus benghalensis* MORACEAE)	Root
	Golden shower (*ratcha phruek* ราชพฤกษ์, *Cassia fistula* LEGUMINOSAE)[33]	Root
	Manila tamarind (*makham thet* มะขามเทศ, *Pithecellobium dulce* LEGUMINOSAE)	Root
Three Medicines with Ambrosial Effect (*trisuraphon* ตรีสุรผล)[34]	Samunlawaeng สมุลแว้ง (*Temmodaphne thailandica* LAURACEAE)	—
	Fragrant heartwood (*nuea mai* เนื้อไม้)[35]	—
	God's tree (*thepphatharo* เทพทาโร, *Cinnamomum parthenoxylon*, syn. *Cinnamomum porrectum* LAURACEAE)	—

Name	Individual Medicinal Components	Part Used
Three Remedies for the Elements (*triphonthat* ตรีผลธาตุ)	Zerumbet ginger (*kathue* กะทือ, *Zingiber zerumbet* ZINGIBERACEAE)	Root
	Cassumunar ginger (*phlai* ไพล, *Zingiber cassumunar* ZINGIBERACEAE)	Root
	Lemongrass (*takhrai* ตะไคร้, *Cymbopogon citratus* GRAMINEAE)[36]	Root
Three Remedies for Having an Effect on Combined Disease (*trisannibatphon* ตรีสันนิบาตผล)	Long pepper (*di pli* ดีปลี, *Piper longum* PIPERACEAE)	—
	Thai holy basil (*kaphrao* กะเพรา, *Ocimum tenuiflorum*, syn. *Ocimum sanctum* LABIATAE)	Root
	Black pepper (*phrik thai* พริกไทย, *Piper nigrum* PIPERACEAE)	Root
Three Medicines of Fragrant Aroma (*trikansawat* ตรีกันสวาต)	Bastard cardamom (*reo yai* เร่วใหญ่, *Amomum xanthiodes* ZINGIBERACEAE)	Fruit
	Nutmeg (*chan* จันทน์, *Myristica fragrans* MYRISTICACEAE)[37]	Fruit
	Clove (*kanphlu* กานพลู, *Syzygium aromaticum*, syn. *Eugenia caryophyllus* MYRTACEAE)	—
Three Black Poison Treatments (*trikalaphit* or *trikanlaphit* ตรีกาฬพิษ)	Finger root (*krachai* กระชาย, *Boesenbergia rotunda* ZINGIBERACEAE)[38]	Root
	Galangal (*kha* ข่า, *Alpinia galanga* syn. *Languas galanga* ZINGIBERACEAE)	Root
	Thai holy basil (*kaphrao* กะเพรา, *Ocimum tenuiflorum*, syn. *Ocimum sanctum* LABIATAE)[39]	Root
Three Celestial Flavors (*trithipphayarot* ตรีทิพยรส)[40]	Costus root (*kot kraduk* โกฐกระดูก, *Saussurea lappa* ASTERACEAE)	—
	Kalamphak กะลำพัก (*Euphorbia antiquorum* EUPHORBIACEAE)	—
	Khondok ขอนดอก (*Asclepias gigantea* APOCYNACEAE)	—
Three Insightful Flavors (*triyannarot* ตรีญาณรส)	Betelnut palm (*mak* หมาก, *Areca catechu* ARECACEAE)	—
	Neem (*sadao* สะเดา, *Azadirachta indica* MELIACEAE)	Root
	Guduchi (*boraphet* บอระเพ็ด, *Tinospora crispa* MENISPERMACEAE)	Vine

Name	Individual Medicinal Components	Part Used
Three Flawless Diamonds (*triphetsamakhun* ตรีเพชรสมคุณ)	Aloe (*wan hang chorakhe* ว่านหางจรเข้, *Aloe vera* XANTHORRHOEACEAE)	—
	Golden shower (*ratcha phruek* ราชพฤกษ์, *Cassia fistula* LEGUMINOSAE)	Pod or hull
	Rong thong รงทอง (*Garcinia acuminata* GUTTIFERAE)	—
Three Medicines that Cut What is Vile (*trichinthalamaka* ตรีฉินทลามกา)	Medicinal rhubarb (*kot nam tao* โกฐน้ำเต้า, *Rheum palmatum* POLYGONACEAE)	—
	Haritaki (*samo apphaya* สมออัพพยา, *Terminalia chebula* COMBRETACEAE)	—
	Rong thong รงทอง (*Garcinia acuminata* GUTTIFERAE)	—
Three Golden Filaments (*trikesonmat* ตรีเกษรมาศ)	Fin ton ฝิ่นต้น (*Jatropha multifida* EUPHORBIACEAE)	Bark
	Lotus (*bua luang* บัวหลวง, *Nelumbo nucifera* NELUMBONACEAE)	Pollen
	Bael tree (*matum* มะตูม, *Aegle marmelos* RUTACEAE)	Fruit, unripe
Three Eternal Things (*tri-amarit* ตรีอมฤต)	Hog plum (*makok* มะกอก, *Spondias pinnata* ANACARDIACEAE)	Root
	Banana, unripe (*kluay* กล้วยตีบ, *Musa* sp. MUSACEAE)	Root
	Kadom กะดอม (*Gymnopetalum cochinchinensis* CUCURBITACEAE)	Root
Three Lineages Wisdom (*trisattakula* ตรีสัตกุลา)	Black cumin (*thian dam* เทียนดำ, *Nigella sativa* RANUNCULACEAE)	—
	Coriander (*phak chi la* ผักชีลา, *Coriandrum sativum* UMBELLIFERAE)[41]	—
	Ginger, fresh (*khing sot* ขิงสด, *Zingiber officinale* ZINGIBERACEAE)	—
Three Medicines for Oil, Sebum or Lymph (*trithurawasa* ตรีทุรวสา)	Horapha thet โหรพาเทศ (*Ocimum* sp. LABIATAE)[42]	Seed
	Cardamom (*krawan* กระวาน, *Amomum testaceum* ZINGIBERACEAE)	Fruit
	Ratchadat ราชดัด (*Brucea amarissima* SIMAROUBACEAE)	Fruit

Name	Individual Medicinal Components	Part Used
Three Things for Having an Effect on Mucus (*trisemhaphon* ตรีเสมหผล)	Wild pepper (*cha phlu* ช้าพลู, *Piper sarmentosum* PIPERACEAE)	Fruit
	Long pepper (*di pli* ดีปลี, *Piper longum* PIPERACEAE)	Root
	Crab's eye vine (*maklam khruea* มะกล่ำเครือ, *Abrus precatorius* LEGUMINOSAE)	Root
Three Things for Having an Effect on Bile (*tripitaphon* ตรีปิตผล)	Chetta mun thet เจตมูลเทศ (*Plumbago* sp. PLUMBAGINACEAE)	—
	Thai holy basil (*kaphrao* กะเพรา, *Ocimum tenuiflorum*, syn. *Ocimum sanctum* LABIATAE)	Root
	Phak phaeo daeng ผักแพวแดง (*Iresine herbstii* AMARANTHACEAE)	—
Three Things for Having an Effect on Wind (*triwataphon* ตรีวาตผล)	Sakhan สะค้าน (*Piper interruptum* PIPERACEAE)	Fruit
	Galangal (*kha* ข่า, *Alpinia galanga* syn. *Languas galanga* ZINGIBERACEAE)	Root
	Black pepper (*phrik thai* พริกไทย, *Piper nigrum* PIPERACEAE)	Root

[...]

Four Entities Group

Name	Individual Medicinal Components	Part Used
Four Medicines for Treating the Elements at Different Times (*chatukanthat* จตุกาลธาตุ)	Calamus (*wan nam* ว่านน้ำ, *Acorus calamus* ARACEAE)	—
	Plumbago (*chetta mun phloeng* เจตมูลเพลิง, *Plumbago* sp. PLUMBAGINACEAE)	Root
	Khaeklae แคแกล (*Dolichandrone serrulata* BIGNONIA-CEAE)[43]	Root
	Pagoda flower (*nom sawan* นมสวรรค์, *Clerodendrum paniculatum* VERBENACEAE)	Root
Four Celestial Perfumes (*chatu thip khantha* จตุทิพคันธา)	Licorice (*cha-em thet* ชะเอมเทศ, *Glycyrrhiza glabra* LEGUMINOSAE)	Root
	Crab's eye vine (*maklam khruea* มะกล่ำเครือ, *Abrus precatorius* LEGUMINOSAE)	Root
	Bullet wood (*phikun* พิกุล, *Mimusops elengi* SAPOTACEAE)	Flower
	Ginger (*khing khraeng* ขิงแครง, *Zingiber officinale* ZINGIB-ERACEAE)[44]	—
Four Fruits for Treating the Elements (*chatu phala thika* จตุผลาธิกะ)	Haritaki (*samo apphaya* สมออัพพยา, *Terminalia chebula* COMBRETACEAE)	Fruit
	Bibhitaki (*samo phiphek* สมอพิเภก, *Terminalia bellerica* COMBRETACEAE)	Fruit
	Amalaki (*makham pom* มะขามป้อม, *Phyllanthus emblica* PHYLLANTHACEAE)	Fruit
	Samo thet สมอเทศ (*Terminalia* sp. COMBRETACEAE)	Fruit
Four Medicines for Having an Effect on Wind (*chatu wata phon* จตุวาตผล)	Ginger (*khing* ขิง, *Zingiber officinale* ZINGIBERACEAE)	Root
	Kalamphak กะลำพัก (*Euphorbia antiquorum* EUPHORBIA-CEAE)	—
	Cinnamon (*opchoei thet* อบเชยเทศ, *Cinnamomum verum*, syn. *Cinnamomum zeylanicum* LAURACEAE)	—
	Sichuan lovage (*kot hua bua* โกฐหัวบัว, *Ligusticum wallichii* UMBELLIFERAE)	—

Five Entities Group

Name	Individual Medicinal Components	Part Used
Five Families (*benchakun* เบญจกูล)	Wild pepper (*cha phlu* ช้าพลู, *Piper sarmentosum* PIPERACEAE)	Root
	Sakhan สะค้าน (*Piper interruptum* PIPERACEAE)	Vine
	Long pepper (*di pli* ดีปลี, *Piper longum* PIPERACEAE)	Fruit[45]
	Ginger (*khing* ขิง, *Zingiber officinale* ZINGIBERACEAE)	Rhizome
	Plumbago (*chetta mun phloeng* เจตมูลเพลิง, *Plumbago* sp. PLUMBAGINACEAE)	Root
Five Families Having an Effect on the Elements (*benchakun phon that* เบญจกูลผลธาตุ)	Umbrella plant (*kokrangka* กกรังกา, *Cyperus alternifolius* CYPERACEAE or *Cyperus digitatus* CYPERACEAE)	Root
	Nut grass (*haeo mu* แห้วหมู, *Cyperus rotundus* CYPERACEAE)	Bulb[46]
	Ya channakat หญ้าชันกาด (*Panicum repens* GRAMINEAE)	Bulb
	Pro เปราะ (*Kaempferia* sp. ZINGIBERACEAE)	Bulb
	Tao kiat เต่าเกียด (*Homalomena truncata* ARACEAE)	Bulb
Five Small Roots (*bencha mun noi* เบญจมูลน้อย)	Ya klet hoi หญ้าเกล็ดหอย (*Desmodium triflorum* PAPILIONOIDEAE)	—
	Ya klet hoi หญ้าเกล็ดหอย (*Hydrocotyle sibthorpioides* UMBELLIFERAE)	—
	Castor oil plant (*rahung daeng* ระหุ่งแดง, *Ricinus communis* EUPHORBIACEAE)[47]	Root
	Cockroach berry (*makhuea khuen* มะเขือขื่น, *Solanum aculeatissimum* SOLANACEAE)	Root
	Ma-uek มะอึก (*Solanum stramonifolium* SOLANACEAE)	Root
Five Large Roots (*bencha mun yai* เบญจมูลใหญ่)	Bael tree (*matum* มะตูม, *Aegle marmelos* RUTACEAE)	Root
	Longan (*lamyai* ลำใย, *Dimocarpus longan* SAPINDACEAE)	Root
	Pheka เพกา (*Oroxylum indicum* BIGNONIACEAE)	Root
	Khaeklae แคแกล (*Dolichandrone serrulata* BIGNONIACEAE)	Root
	Khatlin คัดลิ้น (*Walsura trichostemon* MELIACEAE)[48]	Root
Ten Roots (*thatsa mun yai* ทัศมูลใหญ่)	Collection of "Five Small Roots" and "Five Large Roots" put together	—

Name	Individual Medicinal Components	Part Used
Five Lightning Bolts (*bencha lok wichian* เบญจโลกวิเชียร) [49]	Maduea uthumphon มะเดื่ออุทุมพร (*Ficus glomerata* or *Ficus racemosa* MORACEAE)	Root
	Khon tha คนทา (*Harrisonia perforata* SIMAROUBACEAE)	Root
	Thao yai mom ท้าวยายม่อม (*Clerodendrum petasites* LABIATAE or *Tacca leontopetaloides* TACCACEAE)	Root
	Ya nang หญ้านาง (*Tiliacora triandra* MENISPERMACEAE) [50]	Root
	Ching chi ชิงชี่ (*Capparis micracantha* CAPPARIDACEAE)	Root
Five Refreshing Things (*bencha lo thi ka* เบญจโลธิกะ)	Chan daeng จันทน์แดง (*Dracaena loureiri* AGAVACEAE)	—
	Chan khao จันทน์ขาว (*Tarenna hoaensis* RUBIACEAE)	—
	Chan chamot จันทน์ชะมด (*Aglaia pyramidata* MELIACEAE)	—
	Bat flower (*neraphusi* เนระพูสี, *Tacca chantrieri* TACCACEAE)	—
	Mahasadam มหาสดำ (*Cyathea podophylla* CYATHEACEAE)	—

Seven Entities Group

Name	Individual Medicinal Components	Part Used
Seven Antlers or Horns (*satta khao* สัตตเขา)	Water buffalo (*khwai* ควาย)	Horn
	Sumatran serow (*lian pha* เลียงผา, *Capricornis Sumatraensis*)	Horn
	Deer (*kwang* กวาง)	Antler
	Cow (*wua* วัว)	Horn
	Bison (*kathing* กะทิง)	Horn
	Goat (*phae* แพะ)	Horn
	Sheep (*kae* แกะ)	Horn
[Things for Treating] Urinary Disease[51] (*parameha* ปรเมหะ)	Konpit ก้นปิด (*Stephania hernandifolia* MENISPERMACEAE)	Stem
	Indian nettle (*tamyae tuaphu* ตำแยตัวผู้, *Acalypha indica* EUPHORBIACEAE)	—
	Tamyae tuamia ตำแยตัวเมีย (*Laportea interrupta* URTICACEAE)	—
	Cardamom (*krawan* กระวาน, *Amomum testaceum* ZINGIBERACEAE)	Fruit
	Costus root (*kot kraduk* โกฐกระดูก, *Saussurea lappa* ASTERACEAE)	—
	Rak thet รักเทศ (*Gluta* sp. ANACARDIACEAE)	Fruit
	"Three Fruits"[52] without seed	—

Nine Entities Group

Name	Individual Medicinal Components	Part Used
Nine Teeth (*naowa khiao* เนาวเขี้ยว)	Hog (*sukon* สุกร)	Tusk
	Bear (*mi* หมี)	Fang
	Tiger (*suea* เสือ)	Fang
	Rhinoceros (*raet* แรด)	Horn
	Elephant (*chang* ช้าง)	Tusk
	Wolf (*sunak pa* สุนัขป่า)	Fang
	Manatee (*pla phayun* ปลาพะยูน)	Tusk
	Crocodile (*chorakhe* จรเข้)	Tooth
	Sumatran serow (*lian pha* เลียงผา, *Capricornis Sumatraensis*)	Tooth

Ten Entities Group

Name	Individual Medicinal Components	Part Used
Ten Families with Effect (*thosa kula phon* ทศกุลาผล)	"Small cardamom" (*reo noi* เร่วน้อย, *Amomum villosum* ZINGIBERACEAE)	Fruit
	Bastard cardamom (*reo yai* เร่วใหญ่, *Amomum xanthiodes* ZINGIBERACEAE)	Fruit
	Coriander (*phak chi la* ผักชีลา, *Coriandrum sativum* UMBELLIFERAE)	Fruit
	Water celery (*phakchi lom* ผักชีล้อม, *Oenanthe javanica* APIACEAE)	Fruit
	Licorice (*cha-em thet* ชะเอมเทศ, *Glycyrrhiza glabra* LEGUMINOSAE)	—
	"Thai licorice" (*cha-em thai* ชะเอมไทย, *Albizia myriophylla* LEGUMINOSAE)[53]	—
	Amber (*aphan thong* อาพันทอง)	—
	Ambergris (*aphan khi pla* อาพันขี้ปลา)	—
	Cinnamon (*opchoei thet* อบเชยเทศ, *Cinnamomum verum*, syn. *Cinnamomum zeylanicum* LAURACEAE)	—
	"Thai cinnamon" (*opchoei thai* อบเชยไทย, *Cinnamomum bejolghota* or *Cinnamomum iners* LAURACEAE)	—

Additional Groups

Name	Individual Medicinal Components	Part Used
Five Metals (*bencha loha* เบญจโลหะ)[54]	Bastard teak (*thong kwao* ทองกวาว, *Butea monosperma* LEGUMINOSAE)	Root
	Thong lang nam ทองหลางน้ำ	Root
	Thong lang bai mon ทองหลางใบมน (*Erythrina suberosa* LEGUMINOSAE)	Root
	Snake jasmine (*thong phan chang* ทองพันชั่ง, *Rhinacanthus nasutus* ACANTHACEAE)	Root
	Coral tree (*thong long* ทองโหลง, *Erythrina fusca* LEGUMINOSAE)	Root
Seven Metals (*satta loha* สัตตโลหะ)	The "Five Metals," plus two additional items:	—
	Winter squash (*fak thong* ฟักทอง, *Cucurbita moschata* CUCURBITACEAE)	Root
	Painted copper leaf (*bai ngoen* ใบเงิน, *Acalypha wilkesiana* EUPHORBIACEAE)[55]	Root
Nine Metals (*naowa loha* เนาวโลหะ)	The "Seven Metals," plus two additional items:	—
	Thong khruea ทองเครือ (*Butea superba* LEGUMINOSAE)	Stem
	Champa thong จำปาทอง (*Alangium kurzii* ALANGIACEAE)	—
Five *kot* (*bencha kot* เบญจโกฐ)	Sichuan lovage (*kot hua bua* โกฐหัวบัว, *Ligusticum wallichii* UMBELLIFERAE)	—
	Kot so โกฐสอ (*Angelica dahurica* UMBELLIFERAE)	—
	Kot khamao โกฐเขมา (*Atractylodes lancea* ASTERACEAE)	—
	Angelica (*kot chiang* โกฐเชียง, *Angelica sinesis* UMBELLIFERAE)	—
	Sweet wormwood (*kot chula lampha* โกฐจุฬาลัมพา, *Artemisia annua* COMPOSITAE)	—
Seven *kot* (*satta kot* สัตตโกฐ)	The "Five *kot*," plus two additional items:	—
	Costus root (*kot kraduk* โกฐกระดูก, *Saussurea lappa* ASTERACEAE)	—
	Kot kan phrao โกฐก้านพร้าว (*Picrorhiza kurroa* SCROPHULARIACEAE)	—

Name	Individual Medicinal Components	Part Used
Nine *kot* (*naowa kot* เนาว โกฐ)	The "Seven *kot*," plus two additional items:	—
	Kot phung pla โกฐพุงปลา (*Dischidia rafflesiana* ASCLEPIA-DACEAE)	—
	Kot chada mangsi โกฐชฎามังสี (*Nardostachys jatamansi* VALERIANACEAE)	—
Special *kot* (*kot phiset* โกฐพิเศษ)	The "Nine *kot*," plus three additional items:	—
	Nux-vomica (*kot kakling* โกฐกะกลิ้ง, *Strychnos nux-vomica* LOGANIACEAE)[56]	—
	Pellitory (*kot kakkra* โกฐกักกรา, *Anacyclus pyrethrum* ASTERACEAE)	—
	Medicinal rhubarb (*kot nam tao* โกฐน้ำเต้า, *Rheum palmatum* POLYGONACEAE)	—
Five *thian* (*thian thang ha* เทียนทั้ง ๕)	Black cumin (*thian dam* เทียนดำ, *Nigella sativa* RANUNCU-LACEAE)	—
	Garden cress seed (*thian daeng* เทียนแดง, *Lepidium sativum* CRUCIFERAE)	—
	Cumin (*thian khao* เทียนขาว, *Cuminum cyminum* UMBEL-LIFERAE)	—
	Fennel (*thian khao plueak* เทียนข้าวเปลือก, *Foeniculum vulgare* UMBELLIFERAE)	—
	Dill (*thian ta takkataen* เทียนตาตั๊กแตน, *Anethum graveolens* UMBELLIFERAE)	—
Seven *thian* (*thian thang chet* เทียนทั้ง ๗)	The "Five *thian*," plus two additional items:	—
	Ajowan (*thian yaowaphani* เทียนเยาวพานี *Trachyspermum ammi* UMBELLIFERAE)[57]	—
	Anise (*thian sattabut* เทียนสัตตบุษย์, *Pimpinella anisum* UMBELLIFERAE)	—
Nine *thian* (*thian thang kao* เทียนทั้ง ๙)	The "Seven *thian*," plus two additional items:	—
	Caraway (*thian ta kop* เทียนตากบ, *Carum carvi* UMBELLIF-ERAE)	—
	Psyllium (*thian klet hoi* เทียนเกล็ดหอย, *Plantago ovata* PLANTAGINACEAE)	—

Name	Individual Medicinal Components	Part Used
Special *thian* (*thian phiset* เทียนพิเศษ)	The "Nine *thian*," plus three additional items:	—
	Thian lot เทียนหลอด (*Vernonia anthelmintica* COMPOSITAE)[58]	—
	Thian khom เทียนขม (*Foeniculum* sp. UMBELLIFERAE)	—
	Thian klaep เทียนแกลบ (*Foeniculum* sp. UMBELLIFERAE)	—
Five Lotuses (*bua nam thang ha* บัวน้ำทั้ง ๕)	Sattabut สัตตบุษย์ (*Nelumbo* sp. NELUMBONACEAE)	—
	Sattaban สัตตบรรณ (*Nymphaea* sp. NYMPHAEACEAE)	—
	Lin chong ลินจง (*Nymphaea* sp. NYMPHAEACEAE)	—
	Chong konlani จงกลนี (*Nymphaea lotus* NYMPHAEACEAE)	—
	Nilubon นิลุบล (*Nymphaea cyanea* NYMPHAEACEAE)	—
Special Lotuses (*bua phiset* บัวพิเศษ)	Bua luang khao บัวหลวงขาว (*Nelumbo* sp. NELUMBONACEAE)	—
	Bua luang daeng บัวหลวงแดง (*Nelumbo* sp. NELUMBONACEAE)	—
	Sattabongkot khao สัตตบงกชขาว (*Nelumbo* sp. NELUMBONACEAE)	—
	Sattabongkot daeng สัตตบงกชแดง (*Nelumbo* sp. NELUMBONACEAE)	—
	Bua phuean บัวเผื่อน (*Nymphaea nouchali* NYMPHAEACEAE)	—
	Bua khom บัวขม (*Nymphaea* sp. NYMPHAECEAE)	—
Five *hora* (*hora thang ha* โหราทั้ง ๕)[59]	Hora amarit โหราอมฤต	—
	Hora miksingkhli โหรามิกสิงคลี	—
	Hora thao sunak โหราเท้าสุนัก	—
	Hora bon โหราบอน (*Balanophora abbreviata* BALANOPHORACEAE)	—
	Monkshood (*hora dueai kai* โหราเดือยไก่, *Aconitum carmichaeli* RANUNCULACEAE)	—

Name	Individual Medicinal Components	Part Used
Special *hora* (*hora phiset* โหราพิเศษ)	Hora phak kut โหราผักกูด (*Microlepia speluncae* DENNSTAEDTIACEAE)	—
	Hora khao niao โหราข้าวเหนียว	—
	Hora khao nuea โหราเขาเนื้อ (*Diplazium dilatatum* ATHYRIACEAE)	—
	Hora khao krabue โหราเขากระบือ (*Microlepia platyphylla* DENNSTAEDTIACEAE)	—
	Hora bai klom โหราใบกลม	—
	Hora mahura โหรามหุรา	—
Five Salts (*kluea thang ha* เกลือทั้ง ๕)[60]	Salt mixed with milk *kluea sin thao* เกลือสินเธาว์ [61]	—
	Salt mixed with honey *kluea phik* เกลือพิก	—
	Salt mixed with alcohol *kluea wik* เกลือวิก	—
	Salt mixed with sesame oil *kluea fong* เกลือฟอง	—
	Salt mixed with cow urine *kluea samutthari* เกลือสมุทรี	—
Special Salts (*kluea phiset* เกลือพิเศษ)	A type of salt[62] *kluea sunchara* เกลือสุญจระ	—
	A type of salt *kluea yaowa kasa* เกลือยาวกาสา	—
	A type of salt *kluea withu* เกลือวิทู	—
	A type of salt *kluea dang khali* เกลือด่างคะลี	—
	Uric acid salt *kluea katang* เกลือกะตัง	—
	Sea salt *kluea samut* เกลือสมุทร	—
	A type of salt *kluea suwasa* เกลือสุวสา	—

These groups of Multiple Medicinal Ingredients must include all of the ingredients each time they are used. The names of the groups are like shorthand to save time by just having a single name [for multiple ingredients]. Those who study the topic of medicine must learn and remember the names and categories of these Medicinal Ingredients. Then, if a text refers to a medicine such as "Three Pungents" or "Five Metals," and you don't know exactly what it consists of, you can look in the texts *Khamphi sapphakhun* and *Khamphi samutthan winitchai,* accordingly.

3.4. Methods for Compounding Medicine

1. Medicine that has been pounded into a powder, then rolled and formed into a tablet to swallow.
2. Medicine that has been pounded into a powder, then ground into fine powder to be dissolved in a liquid vehicle[63] to drink.
3. Medicine chopped into pieces and put into a pot[64] full of water. Boil and drink only the water.
4. Pickled herbs soaked for a short time with brine or spirits. Decant the liquid for drinking.
5. Medicine soaked in alcohol. Alcohol is dripped drop by drop into water and then consumed.
6. Medicine burned into charcoal. Take the ash, immerse it in water, and decant the water for drinking.
7. Medicine burned or dry-roasted until charred, pounded into powder, and ground very finely. Dissolved in various liquid vehicles.
8. Distilled medicine refined by capturing steam, i.e. distilled spirits. Drink only distillate.
9. Medicine that has been mixed, wrapped in a cloth, then loaded into small box to be used for inhaling.
10. Medicine that has been mixed, pounded into a fine powder, then placed in a tube and blown into the nose or throat.
11. Medicine cooked with oil, which is then put into small box and dripped onto a wound.
12. Medicinal preparation heated over fire, the smoke of which is then blown onto a wound or affected area.
13. Medicinal preparation rolled into a cigarette and smoked.
14. Medicinal preparation boiled and then used as a gargle or rinse.
15. Medicinal preparation boiled and used for bathing.
16. Medicinal preparation boiled for soaking.
17. Medicinal preparation boiled for rinsing or flushing.
18. Medicinal preparation boiled for steam or sauna.
19. Medicinal preparation used for a poultice.
20. Medicinal preparation used for rubbing or anointing.
21. Medicinal preparation used as a compress.
22. Medicinal preparation used as a suppository.
23. Medicinal preparation boiled for use as an enema.

[...]

Why must vegetative material, animal parts, and minerals that are Individual Medicinal Components be mixed together? In order to assist one another in becoming medicine that is potent in curing disease, medicinal components must be mixed together in a ratio. If just one thing is used, its potency is not enough to heal illness. It changes into just being food. For example, amalaki (*makham pom* มะขามป้อม, *Phyllanthus emblica*) consumed by itself is just food. It must be mixed according to the methods described above in order to be called a medicine for treating disease.

4. Administration of Treatment

The information in this section is extremely important to be careful about. If it is not really learned and experienced, then it is impossible to be a good doctor. This is because the medicine that is to be given to the patient—all the medicines laid out in the texts as being good for curing disease—would [essentially] be lost. If speaking about the usefulness of medicine for curing disease, the benefits are endless. [However,] the practitioner who does not truly understand a medicinal component and gives it to a patient, if mistaken, can kill the patient. Hence, it said that medicine has endless benefit and is also a punishment of the greatest severity. Therefore, before explaining which medicine cures which disease, the methods of clinical examination must be explained since these methods are an important foundation for doctors in the activity of prescribing medicine. It is just one of many arts within the subject of medicine.

Once it is known what ails the patient, the illness can be treated with the method that will cure it. This is an art form and an important part of being a doctor. The texts support and help the doctor a lot. But, regarding the examination of symptoms, the texts can only describe what the symptoms are, the name of the disease, and so on. The [actual] examination of the patient and diagnosis of the problem is something that doctors do with their own eyes and ears. Caring and listening to the truth is something that is in the doctor's heart. Being thorough is comprised of a combination of research, inquisitiveness, and curiosity, as well as doing the examination and coming to a definitive consensus about the patient being sick with [what illness] and what the reason is for that illness. After getting to the truth of the illness, then an opinion can be formed about the method of treatment.

When this is all understood, then it should be clear that if the examination is not done carefully, then the wrong diagnosis will be made. This is comparable to a person losing sight and walking around without knowing which way to go. If this is the case, then the treatment will be completely wrong from the start. Therefore, it should be obvious that the examination is truly an important part of being a doctor. Doctors who are skillful are so because of this art form—that is, the proficiency in foretelling an illness correctly more often than not. In the case of the examination, the methods can be stated, but how you think is a foundation also. Even if you have a well-reasoned view that is based on inquisitive questioning and careful consideration of all the details, the story of the patient will lead the way and the shrewdness and artfulness of the practitioner must also be relied upon. The activity of laying out such a plan within a text is difficult. The main concepts that form the foundation are explained as follows.

Examination Methods

1. History of Patient

    i. Name?

    ii. Where does the patient live? What is the regional habitat like? Pertains to Geographic Causative Factor.

    iii. Nationality? In order to understand their ideology and behavior.

    iv. Place of Birth? Pertains to Geographic Causative Factor.

    v. Age? Pertains to Age Causative Factor.

    vi. How do they eat? (How do people in their village eat?) For analyzing secondary causes and contributing factors.

    vii. What is their family like? (Ask about parents, children, spouse.) For analysis of hereditary factors.

    viii. What kind of daily behaviors or personal habits do they have. Do they smoke opium, drink alcohol, and so on? For analyzing secondary causes and contributing factors.

    ix. Past diseases and symptoms.

2. History of Disease

    i. When did they fall ill? (The initial day and time.) Pertains to Time and Seasonal Causative factors, as well as the duration of the disease.

    ii. What caused the ailment? (What were they doing before falling ill?) Pertains to contributing factors.

    iii. What were the initial symptoms?

    iv. What was the progression of symptoms?

    v. What course of treatment was followed?

    vi. Symptom variance over time?

    vii. Daily symptoms? (In order to know about the severity of symptoms during the periods of the day.) Pertains to Time Causative Factor.

    viii. Observations of symptoms by medical practitioner at time of examination and how important [these symptoms] are understood to be.

3. Examination of Body

    i. What is their appearance or physique like?

    ii. How is their strength or energy?

    iii. What is their mental or emotional state?

    iv. How is the pain?

    v. How is their pulse running?

    vi. How is their breathing?

    vii. Examine heart.

    viii. Examine lungs.

    ix. Examine tongue.

    x. Examine eyes.

    xi.   Examine skin.

   xii.   Examine the affected area (for example, skin sores, wounds, and so on.).

4. Examination of Symptoms

      i.   Temperature.

     ii.   Perspiration.

    iii.   Bowel movements (both ask and examine).

    iv.   Urine (both ask and examine).

     v.   Food consumption.

    vi.   Voice or sound.

   vii.   Sleep.

  viii.   Internal feeling [of body].

    ix.   Feeling in mouth and throat.

     x.   External feeling [of body or skin].

All of this information must be analyzed, as well as anything else that becomes apparent upon further inspection.

[Diagnosis and Treatment]

Once a sufficient examination is done and an opinion is formed, then a conclusive diagnosis can be made:

    i. What are the patient's symptoms, what is the disease type, what is the name of the disease?

   ii. What is the cause of the disease?

  iii. What is the correct method for treating the disease?

  vi. What are the Properties of Medicine that will effectively treat the disease?

After the examination, then an analysis to form an opinion about the method of treatment is done in the following sequence:

1. Examination of Results

    a. In a person with these symptoms, what is the Causative Factor, and what is the specific aspect of that factor?

    b. In a person born in that region, what is the Geographic Causative Factor, and what is the specific aspect of that factor?

    c. In a person of this age, what is Age Causative Factor, and what is the specific aspect of that factor?

    d. Based on the time of illness, what are the Seasonal and Time Causative Factors, and what are the specific aspects of those factors?

    e. What is the progression of the disease, what is its Causative Factor, and what is the specific aspect of that factor?

In summary, identify the disease: what is Distorted, what is the type of Distortion, and what is the name of the disease?

2. Reason for Symptoms

What is Deficient (*khat* ขาด), Excessive (*koen* เกิน), or Conflicted (*krathop krathang* กระทบกระทั้ง), or exactly what causes the abnormality to surface?

3. Course of Treatment

What type of Medicine (with what type of Properties), how much, to be consumed when, how long? Remedy to be administered following the characteristics of the disease.

    [...]

Endnotes

1   In Pāli, the word used in the text, *nahāru*, is defined as "any sinew or ligament in the human and animal body; a tendon, muscle, nerve" (Chanthaburinarunat 1970, p. 393). The Thai words used in this context are *sen* เส้น and *en* เอ็น.

2   Alternatively, Pleura. The Thai word used in the text, *pang puet* พังผืด, is most commonly defined as fascia, but can also refer to a membrane. The Pāli word used in the text, *kilomaka*, refers to the pleura, the lungs, or the right lung.

3   In Pāli, the word used in the text, *papphāsa*, sometimes refers to the lungs in general and other times specifically to the left lung.

4   Also, Stomach. The Pāli word used in the text, *udariya*, can either refer to undigested food in the stomach or to the stomach itself.

5   Alternate spelling: คูถเสมหะ.

6   Most of the time when a medical text refers to Blood, it is strictly referring to the anatomical substance. Other times, Blood functions almost as an additional Element that contains aspects of all the Elements (particulates in blood being Earth, viscosity of blood being Water, temperature of blood being Fire, and movement of blood being Wind).

7   When referring to *lom*, it means movement in the whole body—muscular contractions, nerve impulses, blood movement, etc.

8   This can be interpreted to mean Fire that causes emotion or fever.

9   Although seemingly similar to terms used in Buddhist or Ayurvedic medicine, the words used here have a different interpretation in TTM than in other systems of medicine.

10 Following the Thai Lunar calendar, with the 1st month occurring approximately in December.

11 The Thai word used in most cases to indicate the specific aspect of a Causative Factor that is contributing to a disease is the word for "ranking" (*phikat* พิกัด). Although absent in this case, it is implied.

12 The second volume, which is essentially a review of all the material presented in the first volume, lists the name of the Rainy Season as *watsana ruedu* วัสสานะฤดู, and provides the specific dates.

13 In this text, Blood is listed as the aspect of the Water Element that is dominant during the phases occurring between 8–32 yrs. However, some teachings may refer to Fire during these phases.

14 This text divides the day and night into four periods and gives these particular time frames. However, other texts may list time frames that are slightly different.

15 For the Second and Third Periods, the Disease-causing Factor listed is the Water Element—specifically Blood and Bile, respectively. Other teachings may refer to Fire during these periods.

16 The 32 Parts of the Body is a traditional way of referring to the body. It is the sum of the Twenty Earth Elements and Twelve Water Elements.

17 The Earth Element does not appear in this list.

18 This is a category of extremely grave diseases.

19 It is implied that beyond simply knowing the name of a disease, medical practitioners must be able to correctly *identify* particular diseases.

20 Given in Vol. 2.

21 The term used here (*no* นอ) is only used to describe the horn of a few animals, and has no English equivalent. It technically refers to a protuberance from the head, such as in rhinocerous.

22 The examples given in the chart are representative of the traditional categories for minerals, which are as follows: 1) minerals extracted from plants, 2) salts, 3) non-metallic, inorganic substances, and 4) metallic substances.

23 The lists given for each of the Three Medicinal Tastes are not meant to be exhaustive, but rather to give some examples of

the types of medicines included in each category.

24 *Kot* is a category of plants, mostly in the Artemisia family. The word *kot* has multiple definitions—i.e., ten-million, belt, or knot-like. The latter may be the most appropriate definition in this case, since these medicinal components all bear a resemblance to something knot-like.

25 *Thian* is a category of plants that are all seed-like.

26 In this context, *chan thet* is referring to sandalwood. However, it is used in other contexts to refer to nutmeg (*Myristica fragrans*).

27 Anything with the Toxic Taste is slightly toxic or toxic if taken in excess. This Taste is used to treat poison and toxins in the body, including toxins arising from Bile, Blood and Mucus. It also treats animal and insect bites, fatigue, Toxic Fever, etc.

28 In the original text, the groupings in this section appear as lengthy lists. Here they have been organized into tables and listed by the name of the group, the individual medicinal components, and the part used, if specified. The individual medicinal components are spelled in Thai as they are in the text, with any alternate Thai spellings listed as footnotes. When, in a small number of cases, I have created a English common name for a plant that has none, I have based this name on a literal translation of the Thai, and have placed the common name in quotations. When the exact species is unclear, I have given the genus name with the abbreviation "*sp.*"

29 Alternatively, from the official dictionary of the Royal Institute of Thailand (p. 431): cardamom–leaf (*krawan* กระวาน, *Amomum testaceum* ZINGIBERACEAE), cinnamon (*opchoei thet* อบเชยเทศ, *Cinnamomum verum* LAURACEAE), and patchouli–root (*phimsen ton* พิมเสนต้น, *Pogostemon cablin* LABIATAE).

30 Haritaki is also known as *samo thai* สมอไทย.

31 Given in Vol. 2.

32 This grouping is also referred to as the "Three Tastes."

33 Golden shower is also referred to as *khun* คูน.

34 The Thai word *phon* ผล can either mean "fruit" in the literal sense, or "effect," as in "the fruit of one's labor." In the context of this grouping, it is referring to an effect.

35 No tree is specified.

36 *Takhrai hom* ตะไคร้หอม is what is actually mentioned in the text. However, this is most likely not a reference to citronella grass (*Cymbopogon nardus*) since it is not usually used as a remedy. I have interpreted this as referring to lemongrass, which is a common medicinal with a similar name and appearance.

37 In this context, *chan* จันทน์ refers to nutmeg. Nutmeg is more commonly known as *luk chan* ลูกจันทน์.

38 The common spelling for finger root is *krachai* กระชาย, although it is spelled in the text *kachai* กะชาย.

39 Alternate spelling: *kraphrao* กระเพรา.

40 Alternatively, from the official dictionary of the Royal Institute of Thailand (p. 430): costus root (*kot kraduk* โกฐกระดูก, *Saussurea lappa* ASTERACEAE), fragrant heartwood (*nuea mai* เนื้อไม้) and "Thai cinnamon" (*opchoei thai* อบเชยไทย, *Cinnamomum bejolghota* or *Cinnamomum iners* LAURACEAE).

41 Commonly referred to as *phak chi* ผักชี.

42 The Royal Institute Dictionary (p. 430) lists sweet basil (*horapha* โหระพา, *Ocimum basilicum* LABIATAE) here.

43 Alternate spelling: *khaetrae* แคแตร.

44 Ginger is normally simply written *khing* ขิง, and it is possible that a particular variety of ginger is meant here.

45 Given in Vol. 2.

46 Given in Vol. 2.

47 Alternate spelling: *lahung* ละหุ่ง.

48 Alternate spelling: *katlin* กัดลิ้น.

49 The word used in the text, *wichian* วิเชียร, translates as lightning or thunderbolt, diamond, or the earthly weapon of Indra. This grouping of medicinal ingredients is also known as "Five Crystals" or "Five Roots."

50 Alternate spelling: *ya nang* ย่านาง.

51 The name of this grouping, *parameha* ปรเมหะ, shares a name with an ancient medical treatise on urinology.

52 See "Three Fruits" in the **Three Entities Group**.

53 Thai common names are not necessarily given on the basis of genus and species. For example, this plant's name contains the word *cha-em,* which is Thai for licorice, not because it is related to licorice (*Glycyrrhiza glabra*), but because it is sweet like licorice.

54 These are plants that have the word for a type of metal, usually gold, in their Thai names.

55 The plant listed in the text is *ton bai thong* ต้นใบทอง. This is most likely a reference to painted copper leaf.

56 Another name for *Strychnos nux-vomica* is *salaengchai* (แสลงใจ). It is also known as "poison nut" or "strychnine tree," and is a source of the poisonous alkaloids strychnine and brucine.

57 Alternate spelling: *thian yaowaphani* เทียนเยาวพาณี.

58 Alternate spelling: *thian luat* เทียนลวด.

59 The word *hora* โหรา is difficult to translate in this context. It can be translated as "astrological," and also "hour." Neither definition particularly relates to these plants or the way they are used for treating disease (for the most part, these plants are toxic and need to be prepared in a special way to lessen the poison). Their use is not very widespread.

60 According to the *Guide to Medical Science* (Ministry of Education, 2006), the "Five Salts" components are prepared using a method that involves mixing sea salt with fresh water in an earthenware pot and boiling until the water evaporates. When cooled, the resulting salt is divided into five groups and mixed with the various ingredients in a ratio of two parts salt to one part liquid. The mixture is then dried again, resulting in the salts listed here.

61 *Kluea sin thao* เกลือสินเธาว์ commonly means "rock salt," but in this context it is used to refer to the salt that is produced through the process described above.

62 No information could be found describing the difference between many of these salts.

63 Vol. 1 states that the fine powder is to be dissolved in "water" (*nam* น้ำ). Vol. 2 uses the word "liquid vehicle" (*namkrasai* น้ำกระสาย). Examples of liquid vehicles include water, rosewater, tea, honey, lime juice, etc.

64 Referring to an earthenware pot (*mo* หม้อ) traditionally used for preparing medicines.

Bibliography

TTM References

The references listed here are the sources that we mentioned in footnotes and that we consulted most frequently for the information presented in this book.

Anderson, Edward F. (1993). *Plants and People of the Golden Triangle: Ethnobotany of the Hill Tribes of Northern Thailand.* Portland, OR: Dioscorides Press.

Aroonmanakun, Wirote (2011). Thai Romanization Software (Version 1.5). Retrieved August 30, 2013 from http://pioneer.chula.ac.th/~awirote/resources/thai-romanization.html

Brun, Viggo and Trond Schumacher. (1994). *The Traditional Herbal Medicine of Northern Thailand.* Bangkok: White Lotus.

Chaichakan Sintorn. (1997). *Traditional Medicine Hospital Handbook for Course in Thai Medicine.* Chiang Mai: Shivagakomarpaj Traditional Medicine Hospital.

Chanthaburinarunat (1970). *Pathanukrom Bali Thai Angrit Sansakrit chabap Phrachao Borommawongthoe Krommaphra Chanthaburinarunat* [Pāli-Thai-English-Sanskrit Dictionary compiled by His Royal Highness Prince Kitiyakara Krommaphra Chandaburinarunath.] Bangkok: Mahamakutrachawitthayalai.

Department of Agriculture (n.d.). *Thabian phan phuet nai prathet Thai* [Registry of Plants in Thailand]. Bangkok: Department of Agriculture.

Faculty of Pharmacy at Mahidol University (2008). *Sapphaet Thai* [Thai Medical Terminology]. Bangkok: Hanghunsuanchamkat saengthiankanpim.

Faculty of Pharmacy at Mahidol University (May 2000). "PHARM Select." *PHARM Database.* Retrieved August 30, 2013 from http://www.medplant.mahidol.ac.th/pharm/search.asp

Jacquat, Christiane. (1990). *Plants from the Markets of Thailand.* Bangkok: Editions Duang Kamol.

McFarland, George Bradley (1944). *Thai-English Dictionary.* Stanford: Stanford University Press.

McMakin, Patrick D. (2000). *Flowering Plants of Thailand: A Field Guide.* Bangkok: White Lotus.

Ministry of Commerce and Communications. (1930). *Some Siamese Medicinal Plants Exhibited at the Eighth Congress of Far Eastern Association of Tropical Medicine.* Bangkok: Botanical Section, Ministry of Commerce and Communications.

Ministry of Education (2006). "Nomenclature Dictionary." In *Phaetsat songkhro* [Guide to Medical Science]. Retrieved from http://thrai.sci.ku.ac.th/node/523

Mulholland, Jean. (1987). *Medicine, Magic, and Evil Spirits*. Canberra: The Australian National University.

Mulholland, Jean. (1988). "Ayurveda, Congenital Disease and Birthdays in Thai Traditional Medicine." *Journal of the Siam Society* 76: 174–82.

National Identity Board. (1991). *Medicinal Plants of Thailand Past and Present*. Bangkok: National Identity Board.

Pecharaply, Daroon. (1994). *Indigenous Medicinal Plants of Thailand*. Bangkok: Department of Medical Sciences, Ministry of Public Health.

Poulsen, Anders. (2007). *Childbirth and Tradition in Northeast Thailand*. Copenhagen: Nias Press.

Research and Development Institute, Government Pharmaceutical Organization. (nd). <http://www. rdi.gpo.or.th> Last accessed in 2003.

Rhys Davids, T.W. and William Stede (1972). *The Pāli Text Society's Pali-English Dictionary*. London: Pali Text Society.

Royal Institute of Thailand (2003). *Photchananukrom chabap Ratchabandittayasathan, pho so 2542* [Royal Institute Dictionary, 2542 B.E.]. Bangkok: Nanmi buk phaplikhechan.

Salguero, C. Pierce. (2007). *Traditional Thai Medicine: Buddhism, Animism, Ayurveda*. Prescott, AZ: Hohm Press.

Saralamp, Promjit et al. (1996–97). *Medicinal Plants in Thailand, Vols. 1–2*. Bangkok: Department of Pharmaceutical Botany, Mahidol University.

School of Traditional Medicine at Wat Phra Chetuphon (undated reprint of 1909 edition). *Wetchasueksa Phaetsatsangkhep, Lem 1–3* [The Study of Medicine, Summary of Medical Science, Vols. 1–3]. Bangkok: Nam akson kanphim.

School of Traditional Medicine at Wat Phra Chetuphon. (1964–1977). *Pramuan sapphakhun ya Thai lem 1-3* [A Collection of the Properties of Medicine, Books 1-3]. Bangkok: Mahamakutratchawitthayalai.

Smitinand, Tem (1980). *Chue Phanmai Haeng Prathet Thai* [Thai Plant Names]. Bangkok: Krom Pamai.

Somchintana, Ratarasarn. (1986). *The Principles and Concepts of Thai Classical Medicine*. Bangkok: Thai Khadi Research Institute, Thammasat University.

Thai Pharmaceutical Committee. (1995). *Thai Herbal Pharmacopoeia*. Bangkok: Department of Medical Sciences, Ministry of Public Health.

Thiangburanatham, Wit (1996). *Photchananukrom Thai-Angrit* [Thai-English Dictionary]. Bangkok: Ruam San.

Thiangburanatham, Wit. (1990). *Photchananukrom rok lae samunphrai Thai* [Dictionary of Disease and Thai Herbs]. Bangkok: Rongphim Aksonphithaya.

Thiangburanatham, Wit. (1990). *Photchananukrom samunphrai Thai* [Dictionary of Thai Herbs.] Bangkok: Rongphim Aksonphithaya.

Traditional Medicine Development Foundation. (2001). *Food For Health.* Nontaburi: Textbook Development Project.

Wutthithammawet, Wut (2009). *Khrueang ya Thai* [Thai Materia Medica]. Bangkok: Silpa Siam.

Wutthithammawet, Wut. (1995). *Saranukrom samunphrai* [Encyclopedia of Herbs]. Bangkok: Odian Store.

Wutthithammawet, Wut. (2004). *Khamphi phesat rattanakosin* [Treatise of Pharmacy of the Current Era]. Bangkok: Wuthikammawet.

Other Herbal Traditions

These references were consulted on a less frequent basis in preparation of the compendium, in order to draw comparisons and make cross-references to other traditions.

Balz, Rodolphe. (1996). *The Healing Power of Essential Oils.* Twin Lakes, WI: Lotus Press.

Frawley, David. (1989). *Ayurvedic Healing: A Comprehensive Guide.* Delhi: Motilal Banarisidass Publishers.

Frawley, David. (1993). *The Yoga of Herbs.* Twin Lakes, WI: Lotus Press.

Grieve, Maud. (1981). *A Modern Herbal.* Eugene, OR: Mountain Rose Herbs. (This book is available online at www.botanical.com.)

Kaptchuk, Ted J. (1983). *The Web That Has No Weaver.* Chicago: Congdon & Weed.

Lust, John. (2001). *The Herb Book.* New York: Benedict Lust Publications.

Miller, Light and Bryan Miller. (1995). *Ayurveda and Aromatherapy.* Twin Lakes, WI: Lotus Press.

Ranade, Subhash. (1999). *Natural Healing Through Ayurveda.* Twin Lakes, WI: Lotus Press.

Reid, Daniel. (1995). *The Complete Book of Chinese Health and Healing: Guarding the Three Treasures.* Boston: Shambhala Publications.

Tierra, Michael. (1998). *Chinese Traditional Herbal Medicine Vol. 1: Diagnosis and Treatment.* Twin Lakes, WI: Lotus Press.

Tierra, Michael. (1998). *The Way of Herbs.* New York: Pocket Books.

Thai History

These references were consulted in the writing of Chapter 1, and are recommended for further reading on the history of Thai medicine and of Thailand more generally.

Coedes, G. (1983). *The Making of Southeast Asia* (Translated by H. M. Wright). Berkeley: University of California Press.

Diamond, Jared. (1999). *Guns, Germs, and Steel: The Fates of Human Societies*. New York: W. W. Norton and Company.

Horner, I.B. (2000). *The Book of the Discipline (Vinaya-Pitaka), Vol. IV (Mahavagga)*. Oxford: Pali Text Society.

Lockard, Craig. (2009). *Southeast Asia in World History*. Oxford: Oxford University Press.

Salguero, C. Pierce. (2007). *Traditional Thai Medicine: Buddhism, Animism, Ayurveda*. Prescott, AZ: Hohm Press.

Terwiel, B.J. (1991). *A Window on Thai History*. Bangkok: Duang Kamol.

Wyatt, David. (2003). *Thailand: A Short History*. New Haven: Yale University Press.

TTM Suppliers and Schools

Where to Purchase Thai Herbs

While one is not likely to find a medicinal Thai herb shop in countries outside Thailand, many edible Thai herbs that have both culinary and medicinal uses can be found in Asian grocery stores in Western countries. In addition, there are many medicinal Thai herbs that can easily be found in Chinese and Ayurvedic medicine supply shops. In addition to these possibilities, when looking for Thai herbs you may try the following suppliers. Please note that we do not guarantee quality of product or service.

THE NAGA CENTER SCHOOL OF
TRADITIONAL THAI MASSAGE AND MEDICINE
United States
www.nagacenter.org

Makes small-batch traditional Thai herbal formulas (with magic).

THAI-HERBS.COM
United States
www.Thai-Herbs.com

Sells Thai herbal compresses as well as bulk herb mix for making your own compresses.

THANYAPORN HERBS
Bangkok, Thailand.
www.thanyaporn.com

Sells many medicinal Thai herbs in capsules and teas. Ships internationally. Most likely it will not say this on the packaging, but generally capsules in Thailand are made from rice, and are therefore vegetarian and vegan friendly.

RAKSA HERBS
Bangkok, Thailand
www.raksaherbs.com

Sells Thai herbal compresses. Ships internationally.

BIO THAI NATURAL PRODUCTS
Italy
www.biothai.it

Primarily sells spa products, but is one of the few European retailers that has Thai herbal compresses and some herbal formulas.

Where to Study Thai Herbal Medicine

A dedicated student may be able to find practitioners in Thailand who will share some formulas or other teachings (especially if the students speaks Thai, or comes with a translator), but this will take effort. A comprehensive program in Thai herbal medicine remains difficult to find if one does not speak Thai fluently.

**THE NAGA CENTER SCHOOL OF
TRADITIONAL THAI MASSAGE AND MEDICINE**
Portland, Oregon, United States
www.nagacenter.org

At present, the Naga Center offers the only in-depth and hands-on curriculum in Thai herbal medicine that we know of in the English language.

Where to Study Thai Herbal Compress Massage

The branch of TTM that is most accessible to non-Thais is the bodywork. Thai massage schools that cater to travelers in Thailand are abundant and easily found with a quick online search. Many such schools include instruction in herbal compress massage. We have listed a few below that are known to place extra emphasis on this practice. The schools and teachers listed here are ones that, at the time of this writing, we know to integrate Thai herbal compress massage into the larger practice and theory of TTM.

BODYMIND THAI
Newington, Connecticut, United States
www.bodymindthai.com

ESCUELA NUAD THAI
Buenos Aires, Argentina
www.escuelanuadthai.com.ar

THE NAGA CENTER SCHOOL OF TRADITIONAL THAI MASSAGE AND MEDICINE

Portland, Oregon, United States

www.nagacenter.org

SACRED ASIA SCHOOL OF ANCIENT THAI MASSAGE

Vancouver, British Columbia, Canada

www.ancientthaimassage.ca

SCHOOL OF THAI HEALING ARTS (SOTHA)

Rome, Italy

www.learnthaimassage.org

SHIVAGO THAI SCHOOL OF TRADITIONAL THAI THERAPY

Edinburgh, Scotland, United Kingdom

www.shivagothaischool.com

THAI MASSAGE SCHOOL OF THAILAND

Chiang Mai, Thailand

www.tmcschool.com

Index by Common English Name

Index by Common Thai Name

This index lists the common thai names of the medicinal substances described in Chapter 6 of this book, with both systems of transcription. Refer to the index of common English names above to find them in the book.

má-kăam-bpôm see amalaki

má-dtoom see bael

má-hăa-hĭng see asafoetida

má-kăam kàek see senna

má kăam see tamarind

má-kam-dee-kwaai see soap nut

má lá gor see papaya

má-lí see jasmine

má-mûang see mango

má naao see lime

ma phráao see coconut

má-rá kiî nók see bitter gourd

má rum see moringa

má yom see otaheite gooseberry

màak pûu màak mia see ti plant

mahahing see asafoetida

makham khaek see senna

makham pom see amalaki

makham see tamarind

makhamdikhwai see soap nut

makluea see ebony tree

makphumakmia see ti plant

makrut see kaffir lime

malako see papaya

mali see jasmine

mamuang see mango

manao see lime

mang kút see mangosteen

mangkhut see mangosteen

maphrao see coconut

mara khi nok see bitter gourd

marum see moringa

matum see bael

mayom see otaheite gooseberry

nám pêung see honey

nám-dtaan bpèuk see palm sugar

nam phueng see honey

namtan puek see palm sugar

nga see sesame seeds

ngaa see sesame seeds

ngèuak bplaa mŏr see sea holly

ngueak pla mo see sea holly

nói nàa see sugar apple

noina see sugar apple

nom see milk

oi see sugar cane

ôi see sugar cane

op-choie see cinnamon

opchoei see cinnamon

pá-yaa yor see snake grass

pàk-bûng see morning glory

phak bung see morning glory

pàk-bûng-tá-lay see railroad vine

phak bungthale see railroad vine

pàk grà chàyt see water mimosa

pàk krâat hŭa waen see paracress

phàk-chee see coriander

phak chi see coriander

phak khrat hua waen see paracress

phak krachet see water mimosa

phaya yo see snake grass

phimsen see borneol

phlai see cassumunar ginger

phlu see betel leaf

phluu see betel leaf

phrik khi nu see mouse pepper

phrik thai dam see black pepper

pim-săyn see borneol

plai see cassumunar ginger

prík-kêe-nŭu see mouse pepper

prík tai dam see black pepper

raang jèut see purple allamanda

rak yai see lacquer tree

rák yài see lacquer tree

rangchuet see purple allamanda

sà-dao see neem

sà-mŏr-pí-pâyk see bibhitaki

sà-mŏr-tai see haritaki

sà-rá-nàe see mint

săan sôm see alum powder

sadao see neem

sàkáan see sakaan

sakhan see sakaan

samo phiphek see bibhitaki

Index by Latin Name

This index lists the Latin botanical names of the medicinal substances described in Chapter 6 of this book. Refer to the index of common English names above to find them in the book.

Cassia alata see candelabra bush
Cassia fistula see golden shower
Cassia tora see foetid cassia
Centella Asiatica see asiatic pennywort
Chloranthus erectus see chicken bone
Chrysanthemum morifolium see chrysanthe-
　　mum
Cinchona calisaya see chinchona
Cinnamomum camphora see camphor
Cinnamomum spp. see cinnamon
Citrus aurantifolia see lime
Citrus hystix see kaffir lime
Citrus maxima see pomelo
Clinacanthus nutans see snake grass
Clitoria ternatea see butterfly pea
Coccinia grandis see ivy gourd
Cocos nucifera see coconut
Commiphora myrrha see myrrh
Cordyline fruticosa see ti plant
Coriandrum sativum see coriander
Crocus sativus see saffron
Cryptolepis buchanani see wax-leaved climber
Cucurbita maxima see pumpkin
Cucurbita moschata see pumpkin
Curcuma longa see turmeric
Curcumin zedoaria see zedoary
Cymbopogon citratus see lemongrass
Cyperus rotundus see nutgrass
Dimocarpus longan see longan
Diospyros mollis see ebony tree
Durio zibethinus see durian
Eryngium foetidum see culantro
Ferula assafoetida see asafoetida
Foeniculum vulgare see fennel
Garcinia cambogia see garcinia
Garcinia mangostana see mangosteen
Gloriosa superba see gloriosa lily
Glycyrrhiza glabra see licorice
Hibiscus sabdariffa see roselle
Illicium verum see star anise
Impatiens balsamina see garden balsam
Imperata cylindrica see woolly grass

Ipomoea aquatica see morning glory
Ipomoea pes-caprae see railroad vine
Jasminum spp. see jasmine
Lagerstroemia speciosa see crepe myrtle
Lawsonia inermis see henna
Ligusticum wallichii see sichuan lovage
Mangifera india see mango
Melanorrhoea usitata see lacquer tree
Mentha spp. see menthol
Mentha spp. see mint
Michelia champaca see champaca
Momordica charantia see bitter gourd
Morinda citrifolia see noni
Moringa oleifera see moringa
Morus alba see mulberry
Musa spp. see banana
Myristica fragrans see mace
Myristica fragrans see nutmeg
Nelumbo nucifera see lotus
Neptunia oleracea see water mimosa
Ocimum tenuiflorum see basil
Orthosiphon aristatus see cat's whisker
Oryza sativa see rice
Pandanus amaryllifolius see pandanus
Papaver somniferum see opium poppy
Phyllanthus acidus see otaheite gooseberry
Phyllanthus emblica see amalaki
Pimpinella anisum see anise
Piper betel see betel leaf
Piper interruptum see sakaan
Piper longum see long pepper
Piper nigrum see black pepper
Piper sarmentosum see wild pepper leaf
Plantago spp. see plantain
Plumbago spp. see plumbago
Potassium aluminium sulfate see alum powder
Psidium guajava see guava
Punica granatum see pomegranate
Pyllanthus niruri see stonebreaker
Quisqualis indica see rangoon creeper
Rhinacanthus nasutus see snake jasmine
Ricinus communis see castor oil plant

Index by Taste

The medicinal tastes are discussed in detail in Chapter 2, and are mentioned repeatedly throughout the book. This index lists medicinal substances by their tastes. Refer to the index of common English names above to find them in the book.

Aromatic Pungent: angelica, anise, borneol, cardamom, cinnamon, clove, coriander, costus root, fennel, lemongrass, mint, nutgrass, nutmeg, star anise

Astringent: alum, amalaki, bael, banana, bibhitaki, cassumunar ginger, coriander, culantro, durian, ebony tree, green tea, guava, haritaki, hanuman prasan kai, henna, honey, lacquer, lotus, mango, mangosteen, myrrh, nutmeg, papaya, pomegranate, tamarind, turmeric, zedoary

Bitter: aloe, amalaki, andrographis, asiatic pennywort, basil, bitter gourd, borneol, calamus, candelabra bush, champaca, chinchona, coriander, crepe myrtle, culantro, durian, finger root, foetid cassia, galangal, golden shower, guduchi, haritaki, hanuman prasan kai, jasckfruit, jasmine, long pepper, moringa, need, papaya, sandalwood, sesame, soap nut, stonebreaker, sugar cane, turmeric, wax-leaved climber, yanaang, zerumbet ginger

Chum: angelica, asafoetida, durian, garden balsam, moringa

Cooling: aloe, borneol, butterfly pea, chrysanthemum, guduchi, ivy gourd, mangosteen, mulberry, pineapple, plantain, railroad vine, snake grass, ti plant, water mimosa, white clay

Fragrant/Cool: angelica, champaca, chrysanthemum, coriander, damask rose, jasmine, kaffir lime, lotus, menthol, myrrh, pandanus, pomelo, rangoon creeper, saffron, sandalwood, sichuan lovage, ylang ylang

Heating: anise, asafoetida, bael, black pepper, calamus, camphor, cassumunar ginger, castor oil plant, durian, ebony tree, gloriosa lilly, honey, mango, moringa, mouse pepper, noni, plumbago, rangoon creeper, safflower, sakaan, sea holly, shallot, tamarind

Mild: angelica, cinnamon, costus root, sichuan lovage

Oily: banana, coconut, costus root, jackfruit,

lotus, milk, moringa, pumpkin, rangoon creeper, rice, sesame, sichuan lovage, sugar apple, ti plant

Pra: camphor, henna

Salty: coconut, oyster shell, sea holly, sea salt

Sour: alum, amalaki, bibhitaki, garcinia, golden shower, haritaki, kaffir, lime, mango, mulberry, otaheite gooseberry, papaya, pineapple, pomegranate, roselle, senna, tamarind

Spicy/Hot: basil, black pepper, clove, durian, finger root, galangal, garlic, ginger, hanuman prasan kai, long pepper, mace, moringa, mouse pepper, onion, sakaan, wild pepper leaf, zedoary, see also Aromatic Pungent

Sweet: anise, bael, banana, basil, bibhitaki, coconut, coriander, culantro, durian, fennel, ginger, golden shower, honey, jackfruit, licorice, longan, mango, mangosteen, milk, moringa, mulberry, palm sugar, papaya, pineapple, plantain, pomegranate, pumpkin, rice, safflower, senna, sesame, sugar cane, wax-leaved climber, woolly grass

Tasteless: cat's whisker, moringa, morning glory, mulberry, purple allamanda, snake grass, ti plant, water mimosa, yanaang

Toxic: betel, camphor, candelabra bush, cassumunar ginger, foetid cassia, gloriosa lilly, marijuana, opium poppy, paracress, pomegranate, rangoon creeper, snake jasmine, sugar apple, sulfur

Index by Ailments

General Index

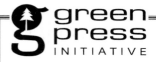

green press
INITIATIVE

Findhorn Press is committed to preserving ancient forests and natural resources. We elected to print this title on 30% post consumer recycled paper, processed chlorine free. As a result, for this printing, we have saved:

11 Trees (40' tall and 6-8" diameter)
5 Million BTUs of Total Energy
958 Pounds of Greenhouse Gases
5,193 Gallons of Wastewater
347 Pounds of Solid Waste

Findhorn Press made this paper choice because our printer, Thomson-Shore, Inc., is a member of Green Press Initiative, a nonprofit program dedicated to supporting authors, publishers, and suppliers in their efforts to reduce their use of fiber obtained from endangered forests.

For more information, visit www.greenpressinitiative.org

Environmental impact estimates were made using the Environmental Defense Paper Calculator. For more information visit: www.papercalculator.org.